Clinical Pharmacology

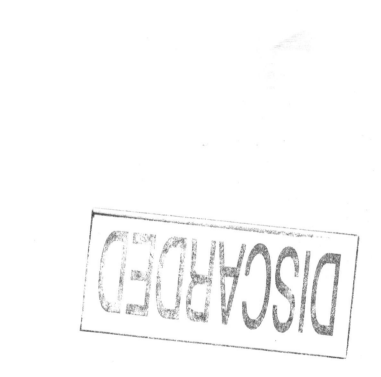

Clinical Pharmacology

Paul Turner
MD BSc FRCP
Professor of Clinical Pharmacology,
St Bartholomew's Hospital, London

Alan Richens
MB PhD FRCP
Professor of Pharmacology and Therapeutics
University of Wales College of Medicine, Cardiff

Philip Routledge
MD MRCP
Senior Lecturer in Clinical Pharmacology
University of Wales College of Medicine, Cardiff

FIFTH EDITION

CHURCHILL LIVINGSTONE
EDINBURGH LONDON MELBOURNE AND NEW YORK 1986

CHURCHILL LIVINGSTONE
Medical Division of Longman Group Limited

Distributed in the United States of America by
Longman Inc. 1560 Broadway, New York,
N.Y. 10036 and by associated companies, branches and
representatives throughout the world.

First edition 1973
Second edition 1975
Third edition 1978
Fourth edition 1982
Fifth edition 1986

ISBN 0-443-03237-8

British Library Cataloguing in Publication Data
Turner, Paul, *1933–*
    Clinical pharmacology. — 5th ed. — (Churchill
    Livingstone medical text)
    1. Drugs   2. Pharmacology
    I. Title   II. Richens, Alan   III. Routledge,
    Philip
    615′.1   RM300

Library of Congress Cataloging in Publication Data
Turner, Paul.
    Clinical pharmacology.
    Includes indexes.
    1. Pharmacology.   2. Chemotherapy.   I. Richens,
Alan.   II. Routledge, Philip.   III. Title.
[DNLM: 1. Pharmacology, Clinical. QV 38 T9501c]
RM300.T86   1986   615′.1   85-24295

Printed in Great Britain by
Butler & Tanner Ltd, Frome and London

Preface to the Fifth Edition

We are delighted that our colleague Dr Philip Routledge has agreed to join us in the preparation of this Fifth Edition. In addition to a thorough revision of the text, we have enlarged Chapter 20 to deal more fully with drugs in the treatment of parasitic infections.

1986   P.T.
                                                                       A.R.

Contents

1

The assessment of new drugs

Until about one hundred years ago, most drugs used in the treatment of disease were derived from naturally-occurring substances of plant or animal origin, for example opium from the poppy, quinine from the cinchona tree and digitalis from the foxglove. In 1827 the glycoside salicin was extracted from the willow bark and in 1874 sodium salicylate was synthesized by Kolbe, introducing the era of synthetic therapeutics. Today the large majority of new therapeutic substances are synthesized in pharmaceutical laboratories and only few are obtained from natural sources.

Synthesis, pharmacological and toxicological testing of new drugs

The development of a new drug occurs in the laboratories of a *synthetic chemist*, and is usually determined by structure activity considerations of related compounds or of endogenously occurring substances with which the new drug is intended to interact. Sometimes, however, completely novel compounds are synthesized in order to evaluate their possible therapeutic effects. Following synthesis, the structure of the new compound and its purity are confirmed by an *analytical chemist*.

It then passes to animal *toxicologists, pharmacologists* and *biochemists* for a series of screening procedures.

(a) Acute studies show the doses necessary to kill a certain proportion of animals, and the mode of death which occurs (e.g. LD_{50} test, which determines the dose that kills 50% of a group of animals).

(b) General pharmacological studies are carried out by routine procedures in isolated organ preparations and in whole animals of different species. These are designed to detect significant activity in one or more systems of the body and to indicate possible mechanisms of action and potential areas of therapeutic value. Care has

1

to be exercised to ensure that preparation of an animal for the experiment does not mask important pharmacological effects. For example, the neuromuscular-blocking activity of suxamethonium (succinyl choline) was missed in early experiments in which its possible ganglion-blocking action was studied in animals paralysed with curare.

(c) Preliminary animal pharmacokinetic studies are carried out to determine the drug's absorption by different routes of administration, its distribution throughout the body compartments and its routes of metabolism. If possible the blood and tissue levels required to produce pharmacological and toxic effects are determined. These investigations are often linked to pharmaceutical studies in which the effects of altering physical and physicochemical characteristics of the drug on its absorption are assessed. Such studies depend on the development of sensitive assay procedures involving gas-liquid chromatography, mass spectrometry, high performance liquid chromatography, radio-immunoassay, or radio-isotope techniques.

(d) Chronic toxicological studies are designed to detect the effect of a drug's long-term administration over a major proportion of an animal's life span. Throughout the study close observation of the behaviour and physiological activities of the animal is carried out, as well as detailed biochemical and haematogical measurements. After death careful histopathological examination of all tissues shows the effects of the drug on various body organs. Studies on two species of animal are usually required, one a rodent and the second non-rodent. It is evident that similar studies must be carried out at each stage on untreated control animals of the same species to determine which apparent abnormalities are due to the drug and which are associated with other age-related, inherited or environmental factors to which the animals are exposed.

(e) Fertility and reproduction studies assumed special importance after recognition of the harmful effects of thalidomide on the developing fetus. These tests can be considered under three headings:

1. Tests of fertility and general reproductive performance in which animals, usually rats, are treated with the new drug before and after mating and its influence on fertility in both sexes, the course of gestation, early and late stages of embryonic and fetal development, lactation and postnatal effects are studied.

2. Teratological studies in which effects of the drug on organo-

genesis are assessed. At least two species are used and the drug is given after mating during the period of organogenesis. Fetuses are carefully examined for visible and skeletal abnormalities, the number of live and dead fetuses recorded, and resorption sites in the uteri and the corpora lutea are examined and recorded.

3. Adverse effects on the mother and offspring in the perinatal and postnatal stages are carried out by treatment during the last third of pregnancy and up to the period of weaning. Observations are made for delayed or prolonged labour, abnormal lactation or maternal care, and direct toxic action of the drug on the young.

Once again, in all these tests, control groups of untreated animals have to be studied in sufficient numbers in order that the effects of the drug may be accurately assessed.

(f) Mutagenicity tests should be carried out before the first administration of a new drug to man. Bacterial tests are commonly employed (e.g. the Ame's test) in which the induction of point mutations is detected in bacterial test systems (e.g. *E. coli* or *Salmonella typhimurium*). These tests appear to be predictors of carcinogenic potential of a compound, and an unequivocal positive result would preclude tests in man until carcinogenic tests had been carried out. Their ability to predict risk of congenital malformations is still uncertain.

(g) Carcinogenicity tests involve administering the drug for a major part of the life span of the species used, examining the tissues thoroughly for malignant changes.

If mutagenicity testing is negative, and if structure-activity relationships give no cause for concern of carcinogenic potential, carcinogenicity tests are not usually required for single-dose or short-term administration of a new drug to normal volunteers or patients.

Studies in man

Drug trials in man may be classified as (a) prophylactic, where a compound's ability to protect against disease is studied, for example antimalarial drugs and vaccines, (b) therapeutic, in which the ability of a drug to treat a disease process already established is assessed, and (c) toxicological, where the emphasis of the investigation is on a drugs toxic rather than therapeutic effects. For example, although digitalis and aspirin have been in therapeutic use for many years, careful studies of the incidence and mechanism of their toxicity are still in progress. This discussion will be limited primarily to therapeutic clinical trials, and these may be subdivided into four phases.

Phase 1. This is a pilot trial, and is generally carried out in normal volunteers. It is designed to answer the following questions about a new drug:

1. What are its characteristics of absorption, metabolism and excretion in man?

2. Are they modified by formulation, prolonged administration or other drug administration?

3. Does the drug possess in man the pharmacological properties shown in animal studies?

4. What is its probable therapeutic ratio, that is, the ratio between the expected therapeutic dose and that producing unacceptable adverse effects? What are its specific dose-dependent adverse effects, and what is the incidence of dose-independent effects? This involves careful assessment of clinical, haematogical and biochemical variables before and after drug administration.

5. What is its mechanism of action?

Phase 1 trials involve depth studies in relatively few subjects. Studies in normal volunteers permit the normal properties of a drug to be assessed and compared with those which are modified by disease.

It is important that those taking part in these, and in later Phase 2–3 studies in patients, should be true volunteers without any coercion. Their informed consent should be obtained after careful explanation of the purpose of the investigation, the procedures to be used and the risks involved. Most institutions in which such research is carried out have set up ethics committees composed of scientific and lay members who review proposed protocols and must give approval before studies may begin. Studies of new drugs in children and in patients with psychiatric conditions require special consideration outside the scope of this book.

Phase 2. This is designed to determine if the new drug possesses the therapeutic effects in patients which were indicated in animal studies and in phase 1 trials in normal human subjects. In many countries, including the United Kingdom and the United States, Phase 2 trials cannot begin until approval is given by government departments on the basis of results of animal and Phase 1 trials.

Initial Phase 2 trials usually begin as 'open' studies, in the sense that the investigator and patients are aware of the nature of the drug administered and of the effect it is likely to produce. If the evidence obtained in these early open studies is suggestive of a therapeutic effect of the new drug, the following questions must be asked:

(a) Has the compound significant therapeutic effects when compared with an identical placebo preparation?

(b) Is the new treatment as good as, or superior to, the best treatment at present avaiable?

An answer to the first question will tell if the drug is really active therapeutically when the bias of the investigator or subject has been excluded. Even if it is active it would not be reasonable to market it commercially if it is inferior to other treatment already available, and this is the reason for the second question. A controlled clinical trial is designed to answer these questions, and usually includes four safeguards against bias: (1) double blind technique, (2) randomization of treatments, (3) matching of patients, (4) well-defined protocol.

Double blind technique

This ensures that neither the investigator nor the subject is aware of the treatment administered. Each treatment, that is the new drug, the standard drug with which it is to be compared and an inactive placebo, are prepared in such a way that they appear identical. Sometimes it is not possible to prepare the new and the standard drugs in identical forms, and it may then be necessary to use two placebos, each identical to one or other of the active compounds, the so-called 'double-dummy' technique. It is important to ensure that the formulation of the standard drug, which is usually a compound in current use, provides the same 'biological availability' as the proprietary preparation. If not, then another error might be introduced, loading the result unfairly in favour of or against the new drug. Biological availability (or bioavailability) in this context means the facility with which a drug can be absorbed from the gastrointestinal tract (or its site of injection if administered parenterally). This may be influenced markedly by the excipient substances, or fillers, present in the tablet or capsule to provide bulk (p. 12), even though they may lack significant pharmacological activity and may not appear to influence the cruder tests of tablet disintegration and dissolution. Another use of the term bioavailability is in the comparison of the blood levels of a drug reached after intravenous administration with those reached after administration of the same dose by some other route (see p. 15). In many situations, it is not ethical to compare a new preparation with a placebo, e.g. in the treatment of a cardiac dysrhythmia or tonic-clonic seizures. Here, comparison with an active treatment prepared in a matching formulation is appropriate.

Randomization of treatments

Controlled trails may be divided into (a) within-subjects trials in which all patients receive each treatment and their responses to each are compared and (b) between-subjects trials where one patient receives only one treatment, the mean responses of each group of patients being compared. The type of trial used depends primarily on the nature of the condition which is being treated. In a chronic condition such as hypertension or rheumatoid arthritis a within-subjects study may be reasonable because a patient may be expected to return to a clinical base line when treatment is discontinued. In conditions which are self-limiting or cyclical in nature, however, such as the common cold or psychiatric states such as anxiety or depression, this assumption cannot be made and so it is not reasonable to compare treatments in the same patient. The advantage of a within-subjects trial is that it usually requires fewer subjects to reach a decision. Randomization of treatments is necessary for two reasons: (a) it avoids observer bias, and (b) it minimizes 'carry-over' effects in within-subjects trails. The administration of one drug may influence the action of subsequent treatments in a variety of ways and so disguise their true effects.

Matching of patients

Among the factors which influence a patient's response to drugs are age, sex, duration and severity of the condition which is being treated. In order to obtain a valid comparison of the activities of various preparations, therefore, and where a between-subjects comparison is necessary, it is desirable to match patients between treatment groups for these various factors. This may prove difficult if the condition is relatively uncommon or tends to occur in one sex more than the other or in one particular age group. A patient's weight may also be an important determining factor in response to a drug. In animal experiments it is usual to administer a drug on the basis of body weight but in therapeutic practice in man this is seldom done except where toxicity is high and dose-related. In fixed-dose studies blood and tissue levels of a drug tend to be higher in lighter subjects, which may produce differences in therapeutic response and toxicity. It is wise, therefore, to match patients for weight whenever possible, or to relate the dose given to their weight.

Before commencing a clinical trial, it is important to define carefully, in writing, the objectives of the trial, the methods to be used in measurement of the appropriate parameters, the details of times of drug administration and various recordings, the statistical comparisons which will be made and by what methods, and the criteria which are considered necessary for inclusion of a subject in the trial and for the assessment of his response to treatment. Once such a protocol has been carefully prepared it should be adhered to throughout the trial.

Statistical analysis

The final stage of a clinical trial is the statistical analysis of the results obtained. Although relatively simple tests such as Chi-squared, Student's *t* and ranking methods may be sufficient where large and obvious differences appear between treatments, more sophisticated methods are available which may show significant differences which are not so readily apparent. Multi-variate techniques of analysis of variance, covariance and dispersion are particularly valuable, for they minimize differences in results due to other factors (such as between-subjects and between-times variations) so that the between-treatment differences are emphasized. These methods are complicated, however, particularly when several different factors are being assessed, and expert help and computer facilities are almost always required.

Although it is desirable to assess the effects of a drug in terms of units of measurement, for example heart rate, blood pressure, body weight or urine volume, there are many types of trial where this is not possible, particularly in investigation of drugs in psychiatry. This may depend on the global judgement of the investigator, as for example, whether a patient is improved or deteriorating. There may also be important ethical reasons for discontinuing a trial as soon as a statistically significant result is obtained, for example in the treatment of malignant conditions. In such circumstances the *sequential trial* may be appropriate. This involves making preferences for one form of treatment against another, either within-patients or between matched patients, and plotting them on a graph prepared from special tables, when the

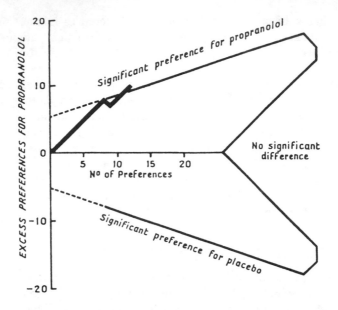

Fig. 1.1 Chart of sequential study for investigator's preferences in a trial of propranolol *v.* placebo in anxiety state. ($\theta = 0.8$, $2a = 0.05$, and $\beta = 0.05$.) (Reproduced from Granville-Grossman K L, Turner P 1966 *Lancet* i, p. 788–790, by kind permission of the editor.)

statistical requirements for significance have been decided. When a line of significance is crossed, either for one drug against another, or of no difference between treatments, then the trial can be discontinued. Figure 1.1 shows such a sequential graph in which propranolol was shown to be significantly superior to placebo in anxious patients after only fifteen preferences had been made, in a double-blind randomized within-patient (cross-over) trial. For most types of investigation of this kind, a probability figure of 5% is usually taken as being significant, so that the chances of obtaining a positive result when in fact it does not really exist are less than 5%, while on the other hand the chances of not obtaining a positive result when one really, exists are also less than 5%.

Strictly speaking, only those statistical comparisons defined in the protocol should be carried out. Some authorities claim that further analysis seeking for significant differences between groups not defined in the protocol is 'data-dredging'. Such analysis may draw attention to factors not previously recognised as important, however, but it is essential that further controlled prospective studies should then be carried out with the objective of confirming that the results of this unplanned analysis are real and not a spurious finding.

Statistical techniques are complex, and wrong conclusions may be reached if an inappropriate one is chosen for a particular problem. For this reason it is wise to include a statistician in the team when planning and carrying out a clinical trial.

Phase 3. Phase 1 and 2 trials have been carried out in relatively few subjects. If they demonstrate therapeutic efficacy and acceptable safety in a new drug, large scale clinical trails are carried out in order to assess its place in wider clinical practice. If results of Phase 3 trials are satisfactory and confirm the drug's therapeutic efficacy and acceptable safety, the pharmaceutical company responsible for it its development may then apply to the regulatory authorities for a product licence which permits its marketing.

Phase 4. Post-marketing surveillance and monitored release Identification of the syndrome of adverse reactions associated with the long-term use of practolol (p. 65) emphasised the importance of close surveillance of large numbers of patients receiving new drugs over a period of many years. Recognition of the practolol syndrome was delayed because it had not previously been associated with other drugs, nor had it been produced in animal models. This demonstrates the necessity to record carefully all clinical events, and the patients' responses to life events such as other illness, pregnancy and bereavement, in sufficient numbers of patients to detect relatively uncommon reactions, over a period of time sufficient to detect long-term adverse effects in the patients or in their offspring. An example of the importance of the latter is the increased incidence of vaginal carcinoma in adolescent daughters of women given stilboestrol early in pregnancy (p. 213).

Several schemes have been proposed to permit identification of patients prescribed a new drug, and regular notification of their clinical progress to central monitoring agencies. Some depend on the assistance of dispensing pharmacists in recording the names of patients prescribed the particular drug. Others seek to exploit the prescription pricing agencies employed in health and welfare services such as the National Health Service in Britain to identify the prescriptions for the drugs under surveillance. Yet others place the responsibility for identifying the patient population on the pharmaceutical company which markets the drug. Every scheme, however, depends for its ultimate success on careful clinical scrutiny of the patient by the prescribing doctor, the meticulous recording of his observations in the patients' documents, and a high index of suspicion that any unexpected clinical event may be associated with a drug's administration.

FURTHER READING

Burley D M, Binns T B 1985 Pharmaceutical Medicine. Edward Arnold, London

2

Factors influencing the action of drugs

Patients differ markedly in their response to drugs. Such differences may be related to variability in drug formulation (pharmaceutical variability) or to intersubject differences. If, for example, a fixed dose of warfarin were prescribed at a dose of 5 mg daily to patients, most would show some degree of therapeutic response. A few, however, would be inadequately anticoagulated whilst others would be excessively anticoagulated and at risk of bleeding. This difference in response is due to two major factors which can vary even in healthy subjects, but are particularly variable in various disease states.

The first intersubject factor is the pharmacokinetic variability between subjects. This term refers to the rate and extent of absorption of the drug, its distribution into the various body compartments, tissue and plasma protein binding, and the rate of metabolism and excretion of the drug. The result of this variability is such that if the plasma level of warfarin were measured, for example, a greater than five-fold difference between subjects would be found even though all were receiving the same dose.

The second factor is the pharmacodynamic variability between individuals, that is the difference between individuals in response to a given concentration of drug at its effector site. A similar degree of variability (about five-fold) in pharmacodynamic responsiveness is seen in healthy patients taking warfarin.

Pharmacokinetics may be termed 'what the body does to the drug', whilst pharmacodynamics refers to 'what the drug does to the body'. Another important determinant of response is what the patient does to the drug. This process is called compliance. Non-compliance is a failure to take the prescribed dose of the drug and is one of the chief reasons for therapeutic failure in the outpatient setting.

PHARMACEUTICAL FACTORS

Many doctors do not realise that when they prescribe a 'drug' the patient actually receives a 'medicine'. Active substance represents only a small proportion of the total weight of an oral solid dosage form such as a tablet or capsule. Similarly, the form of a drug for injection requires solution or suspension in a fluid vehicle of varying complexity. The other constituents of dosage forms are not necessarily 'inert', however, but may play an important part in facilitating or hindering a drug's absorption.

The following are some of the more important factors which are involved in the production of tablets and capsules, and which may influence absorption.

1. Diluents such as lactose or calcium sulphate are used to increase bulk. The importance of these particular diluents in determining the rate of absorption of phenytoin was demonstrated by an outbreak of phenytoin intoxication in Australia when the formulation was changed.

2. Granulating and binding agents, such as tragacanth or syrup are used to assist aggregation of the powder into granules, in order to permit compression into tablets. Bentonite is a naturally occurring mineral consisting chiefly of hydrated aluminium silicate, which is employed pharmaceutically as a binder. It has been shown to adsorb rifampicin rapidly and strongly, and so can significantly decrease the absorption of rifampicin if given simultaneously. It is sometimes used in para-aminosalicylic acid granules in which it aids granulation.

3. Lubricants, such as talc, prevent granule adherence to the tablet punches.

4. Disintegrating agents are incorporated to produce rapid tablet disintegration in the gastrointestinal tract. They include substances such as starch which swell on contact with moisture, substances such as cocoa butter which melt at body temperature, and others such as a mixture of sodium bicarbonate and tartaric acid which effervesce on contact with moisture.

5. Coating materials such as sugar may be used to prevent disintegration before the tablet reaches the stomach or intestine, as well as for cosmetic and identification purposes.

6. Capsules have a gelatin envelope and do not involve granulating excipients. It is a common misapprehension that drugs are released more rapidly from capsule than from tablets; this is not necessarily so.

7. Special formulations employ complex pharmaceutical manoeuvres to control disintegration and dissolution rates, so regulating the rate of a drug's absorption. This has led to the development of sustained release and position release formulations.

8. As well as the foregoing non-drug factors, different manufacturing processes may result in the production of different physical forms of the active drug, and this may influence its rates of dissolution and absorption. The absorption rates of griseofulvin and digoxin, among others, have been shown to be related to particle size.

These matters are relevant to the question of whether generic or brand names should be used in prescribing. The generic or 'approved' name does not necessarily determine the formulation which the patient will receive. Use of the brand name should determine not only the physical form of the drug, but also the excipients and method of manufacture which may influence absorption. Where differences in biological availability of a drug have been shown to be important in patient care, it may be wise to use the proprietary brand name rather than its generic name in prescribing.

PHARMACOKINETIC FACTORS

Absorption

An orally administered drug must pass through the bowel wall in order to enter the bloodstream. This barrier is a complex lipid membrane composed of the walls of the cells lining the bowel. Substances, whether food or drugs, can pass through this membrane in one of four ways:

(a) Passive diffusion, by which the substance passes through the membrane in solution; diffusion is proportional to the concentration difference across the membrane and the lipid solubility of the drug.

(b) Active transport, by which substances (e.g. amino acids) are carried across the membrane by an energy-consuming mechanism, usually against a concentration gradient; some drugs, because of their resemblance to naturally-occurring substances, utilize existing transport systems (e.g. α-methyldopa).

(c) Filtration through pores, which is limited to molecules of small size (e.g. urea).

(d) Pinocytosis, by which small particles are engulfed by cells of the bowel wall. Of these four mechanisms the first, passive diffusion, is by far the most important for drug absorption. Considering then this mechanism in particular, there are a number of factors which will influence absorption:

1. The chemical nature of the drug. Polypeptides are broken down by gastrointestinal enzymes, while benzylpenicillin is destroyed by gastric acid. Large, lipid insoluble molecules for which no active transport system exists are poorly absorbed (e.g. heparin).

2. Formulation (see p. 12).

3. pH. Most commonly-used drugs are either weak acids or weak bases, and these exist in two forms in solution, as undissociated molecules and as ions. The equilibrium between these two forms is determined by (a) the pK value of the drug and (b) the pH of the surrounding medium. At a pH equal to the pK the drug is 50% ionized. At a low pH (i.e. in the stomach) a weakly acidic drug will be mainly in its undissociated form, whereas a weakly basic drug will be largely ionized. In a more alkaline medium (i.e. in the small bowel) the reverse applies. As only the undissociated molecules are appreciably lipid-soluble an acid medium favours the absorption of weakly acidic drugs, while weak bases are better absorbed from the small intestine. A few drugs (e.g. streptomycin and hexamethonium) are strongly basic and their pK values greatly exceed the highest pH reached in the intestine. As these drugs remain ionized throughout the alimentary tract they are very poorly absorbed. Although these general rules explain the behaviour of most drugs, there are some which do not obey these principles for a variety of reasons. For example, sulphaguanidine is very poorly absorbed, not because it remains ionized in the gut, but because its undissociated form is poorly lipid-soluble. Dicoumarol, although highly lipid-soluble, is poorly absorbed because it is relatively insoluble in the alimentary fluid.

4. Gut motility. Most drugs are absorbed from the upper part of the small bowel, and alterations in gut motility can markedly influence drug absorption (see p. 184).

5. Food. Dilution of the drug by food and drink, and the delay in gastric emptying produced by a meal, lead to a slowing of absorption of most drugs. Pain (e.g. in myocardial infarction, migraine or during labour) also delays gastric emptying and it may not be relieved by orally administered analgesics in these circumstances. Unless a drug is irritant to the stomach, it should be taken on an empty stomach. There are, however, some exceptions e.g. griseofulvin is better absorbed after a fatty meal.

6. Liver and bowel wall enzymes. Unless a drug is absorbed

directly into the systemic circulation, as from sublingual administration, it has to pass through the liver via the portal circulation.
Some drugs, e.g. propranolol, lignocaine, chlormethiazole and
oestrogens are extensively metabolized as they pass through the
liver — the so called presystemic or 'first-pass effect'. Induction of
first-pass metabolism can reduce the amount of drug available
systemically.

All these factors influence the 'bioavailability' of a drug, that is,
the extent to which it reaches the systemic circulation.

Drugs may be administered by other routes. They may be given
intramuscularly, although this can sometimes be painful. Some
drugs are rapidly absorbed after intramuscular injection. Peak levels
of lignocaine occur 10 to 15 minutes after intramuscular injection
and absorption from the deltoid muscle is faster than from the
gluteus, probably because of differences in blood flow. In some
cases, however, the absorption is delayed and unpredictable (e.g.
with diazepam) and some drugs (e.g. phenytoin) can crystallise in
the muscle. A few drugs, particularly those with high potency (e.g.
nitrates) can be administered topically. The rate of absorption is
dependent to a large extent on the site of skin used, but attempts
are being made to produce membranes which will control the rate
of diffusion of drugs so that this rate becomes the limiting factor.
Some drugs acting on the airways are given by inhalation or by
nebulisation. It is hoped by this means to achieve high concentrations at the site of action and to reduce systemic toxicity. While
this is to some extent successful, it must be remembered that only
10 to 15% of the drug will enter the airway and the remainder will
be deposited on the buccal mucosa and swallowed. Some agents,
particularly those which undergo extensive presystemic metabolism, may be given sublingually to increase their bioavailability
(e.g. glyceryl trinitrate).

Finally drugs can be given by rectal administration. This can also
to some extent reduce presystemic elimination but the suppository
may be variably retained or have poor and erratic absorption. The
drug in the suppository may also have local adverse effects (e.g.
indomethacin suppositories may cause local bleeding).

Distribution

As a general rule, those drugs which are readily absorbed from the
gastrointestinal tract are freely and rapidly distributed throughout
the body compartments. Diazepam is highly lipid-soluble and is

freely absorbed from stomach or rectum. When injected intra-venously it passes rapidly through lipid barriers into the brain to terminate status epilepticus. It follows that centrally acting drugs, because they have to enter the brain through a lipid membrane, are usually readily absorbed from the gastrointestinal tract. The same drugs, however, can easily gain access to the fetal circulation, and for this reason centrally-acting drugs are the chief offenders in causing fetal abnormalities (e.g. phocomelia caused by thalidomide).

Many drugs are loosely bound to plasma and tissue proteins, and the extent of this binding will affect the kinetics of the drug in question. For a drug showing no appreciable binding the tissues act as little more than a water compartment in which the drug is dissolved. Extensive plasma and tissue protein binding will increase the quantity of the drug which has to be absorbed before effective therapeutic levels of unbound drug are reached at the site of action. A period of many days may be required for equilibration between the body fluids and tissues. A drug which is extensively bound to tissues is said to have a large 'apparent volume of distribution' (Vd). This is a theoretical volume of fluid which would be required to contain the total body content of drug at a concentration equal to the plasma concentration. Nortriptyline is an example of a drug which is extensively tissue bound; its Vd is around 1400 litres. Warfarin, on the other hand, has a Vd of only 7 litres.

Elimination by metabolism and excretion may be delayed when tissue binding is extensive because Vd is one determinant of the plasma half-life ($T\frac{1}{2}$). The greater the quantity of drug requiring elimination, the longer the time to eliminate it completely. The rate of metabolism, as well as the pharmacological effect of a drug, is determined by the concentration of unbound drug in the plasma. However, there are exceptions. When the rate limiting step in metabolism is the delivery of drug to the liver, as it is for propran-olol, plasma protein binding may actually enhance elimination. The former situation is known as 'restrictive' elimination, while the latter is called 'non-restrictive'.

A reduction in concentration of plasma protein may reduce the amount of drug bound, the free drug diffuses in red cells and other tissues and consequently the total plasma concentration (free plus bound) will be lower than expected for a given pharmacological effect. This can occur due to reduced production of binding protein (e.g. hepatic cirrhosis) or because of increased loss (nephrotic syndrome). Renal failure can also reduce the plasma protein binding of some agents due to a reduction in binding affinity of albumin (because of either accumulation of endogenous inhibitors or changes in albumin structure).

In some circumstances, the concentration of the acute phase protein alpha-1-acid glycoprotein increases (e.g. in inflammatory disease and after myocardial infarction or surgery) and this may result in an increase in the plasma protein binding of some basic drugs (e.g. propranolol and lignocaine) which bind to it.

Drugs can compete for plasma protein during sites resulting in a transient increase in effect for drugs with a small Vd. Competition for tissue binding sites has been little studied, but may be in part responsible for the interaction between digoxin and quinidine.

Metabolism

Most drugs administered to man are metabolized by liver enzymes, although some metabolism can occur elsewhere (e.g. in the gastrointestinal tract, lung and blood). Metabolism in the liver occurs particularly with those drugs which are lipid-soluble and therefore can more readily enter the liver cells, whilst their lipid solubility prevents them from being excreted unchanged by the kidney. At first sight it seems surprising that the liver has enzyme systems capable of metabolizing drugs, but the pathways for metabolism are relatively non-specific and protect the individual from potentially toxic agents in the diet. By producing metabolites with increased water solubility the liver enables the kidney to be able to excrete the drug. It has been calculated that if it were not metabolized, a lipid-soluble drug would have a half-life of around 30 days in man and if the drug were reversibly bound to tissues (e.g. thiopentone) and did not undergo metabolism, its half-life would be as great as one hundred years!

Biotransformation pathways can be divided into two major groups. Phase I and Phase II reactions. Phase I reactions are catalyzed by mono-oxygenase enzymes situated in the smooth endoplasmic reticulum of the liver cell. Collectively these are called cytochrome P450 enzymes and they are responsible for oxidation, dealkylation, reduction, or hydrolysis of the drug depending on its molecular structure. Some drugs undergo more than one of these reactions either in turn or separately and the resulting metabolite is often (but not always) biologically inactive. Phase II reactions involve the addition of another generally more water soluble molecule to the drug to form a larger more water soluble and therefore more easily excreted molecule. These are called conjugation reactions and include glucuronidation, sulphation, conjugation with amino acids (such as glutathione) and acetyl CoA (N-acetylation). Although most conjugates are biologically inactive, some acetylated metabolites retain biological activity and may be less water soluble than the parent compound (e.g. N-acetyl procainamide).

The rate of drug metabolism is affected by environmental factors. Drug metabolism is impaired at the extremes of age, i.e. the very young and the very old, and neonates tend to have diminished capacity for both Phase I and Phase II reactions. The half-life of caffeine is 4 days in the neonate compared with 4 hours in an adult and the glucuronidation of chloramphenicol is impaired (this may lead to the serious grey baby syndrome). Nutritional status and constitution of the diet can also affect drug metabolism, although the clinical relevance of these differences is unclear. Some drugs (e.g. phenytoin, barbiturates and rifampicin) and dietary components (hydrocarbons in cigarette smoke and the diet) can induce metabolism primarily by stimulating Phase I reactions (Table 2.1).

Table 2.1   Some drugs causing enzyme induction in man

Anticonvulsants	phenobarbitone
	phenytoin
	carbamazepine
Antibiotics	rifampicin
Anxiolytics and Hypnotics	dichloralphenazone
Miscellaneous	cigarette smoking

Rifampicin, for example, may double the metabolic clearance rate of warfarin. This process takes up to 7 to 14 days to fully develop and when the inducing agent is stopped a similar lag period occurs before the effect wears off. Some agents can impair the metabolism of concomitantly administered drugs (Table 2.2), either by competition between the substrates for the available enzyme, or in a noncompetitive fashion. Cimetidine, although not itself metabolized, may inhibit drug metabolism, for example. Enzyme inhibition generally occurs rapidly after administration of the inhibitor.

Chronic liver disease can be associated with an impairment in drug metabolizing ability. Phase I pathways are affected to a greater

Table 2.2   Some drugs which inhibit drug metabolism in man

allopurinol	isoniazid
amiodarone	ketoconazole
cimetidine	metronidazole
erythromycin	sulphonamides

extent than Phase II conjugation reactions. Thus the metabolism of diazepam is impaired while the metabolism of oxazepam, which is conjugated is much less affected. Unfortunately none of the routinely measured liver function tests gives a clear guide to the degree of impairment of metabolism of the commonly used drugs, although albumin is a rough guide to the severity of reduction in metabolism. If the drug normally undergoes substantial metabolism in the liver, a small change in the ability of the liver to metabolize the drug may markedly affect the amount reaching the systemic circulation since the normally extensive presystemic metabolism will be reduced. The bioavailability of the drug will therefore be much greater than in normal individuals. Propranolol, for example, has much greater bioavailability in patients with chronic liver disease, despite the fact that its degree of absorption from the gut is not different from the normal (i.e. virtually complete).

The metabolism of drugs which are avidly cleared by the liver are limited only by the delivery of the drug to the liver. Hepatic blood flow can fall in heart failure and shock but is also reduced in hepatic cirrhosis due to intra- and extra-hepatic shunting of blood past the hepatocytes. Under these circumstances clearance of the drug will fall when it is given by the intravenous route. The clearance of lignocaine is reduced by approximately a third in patients with heart failure, for example.

Two important metabolic processes are controlled genetically. A difference in activity of hepatic N-acetyl transferase results in three phenotypes with varying ability to acetylate drugs such as hydralazine, isoniazid, dapsone, and procainamide. This is controlled by a recessive gene and 45% of the United Kingdom population are slow acetylators. The remainder are either intermediate or fast acetylators, although the differences between these two groups are fewer than the difference between them and slow acetylators; they are generally grouped together under the fast acetylator phenotype (Fig. 2.1). Over 95% of Canadian Eskimos, but only 18% of Egyptians are rapid acetylators. Slow acetylators have an increased incidence of isonaizid-induced peripheral neuropathy and hydralazine or procainamide-induced systemic lupus erythematosus. They are also less able to tolerate high doses of sulphasalazine in ulcerative colitis. Fast acetylators, however, may be at more risk of isoniazid-induced hepatitis.

Approximately 10% of the British population have a reduction in a specific hepatic monooxygenase responsible for hydroxylation of perhexiline, phenformin, debrisoquine, nortriptyline and some

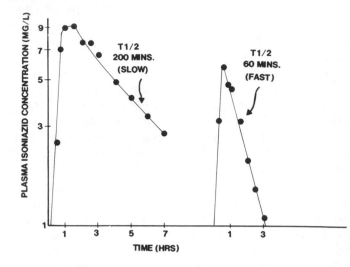

Fig. 2.1 Plasma isoniazid concentrations after 700 mg oral dose in a fast
($T_{\frac{1}{2}} <$ 130 mins) and slow acetylator.

other drugs. These subjects may have an increased risk of developing peripheral neuropathy after treatment with the anti-anginal drug, perhexilene, but the clinical importance of the defect in relation to the other drugs is still unknown.

Excretion

The majority of drugs are excreted in the urine as metabolites of the parent compound but some (e.g. atenolol, chlorpropamide, cimetidine, digoxin, aminoglycoside antibiotics and penicillins) are excreted largely unchanged. Although lipid-soluble drugs may appear in the glomerular filtrate provided they are not appreciably bound to plasma proteins, they readily pass back into the bloodstream by passive diffusion through the proximal tubule. Only when they have been metabolized to more water soluble metabolites will they have difficulty in diffusing back. In addition to undergoing diffusion many acidic and basic drugs are actively secreted into the proximal renal tubule. Two separate mechanisms appear to be responsible for the excretion of bases and acidic drugs and these processes are not generally limited by plasma protein binding. Competition can occur however between compounds. Aspirin can reduce active tubular secretion of another acidic compound, methotrexate, causing a greater risk of toxicity from the latter compound. Finally an active transport system promotes the excretion of digoxin in the distal tubule. It may be affected by other agents such as quinidine, verapamil and spironolactone which will reduce renal digoxin excretion.

Since drugs are passively reabsorbed from the tubular fluid the rate of tubular fluid flow and changes in pH can affect elimination of compounds, particularly weak acids and bases. Normally the urine is slightly acid and this favours the excretion of weakly basic drugs (e.g. amphetamine). This is because weak bases are more highly ionized under acid conditions so that their ability to diffuse back through the lipid membranes of the renal tubular cells is reduced. Further acidification of the urine will demonstrably shorten the action of these drugs while measures to alkalinise the urine may prolong their effects. The reverse applies for weakly acidic drugs (e.g. aspirin, phenobarbitone).

The processes affecting renal drug excretion can be affected by age and disease. The very young have a reduced glomerular filtration rate relative to their body surface area and the active tubular secretory mechanism is also immature. Glomerular filtration rate also falls with increasing age over 40 years of age, although the renal tubular secretory mechanisms appear to be less affected. Renal failure is also associated with a reduction in glomerular filtration rate. Measurement of this or of serum creatinine or blood urea can enable the physician to adjust the dose of drugs for which glomerular filtration is the most important pathway of excretion (e.g. gentamicin and digoxin). It is of less value for drugs like penicillins in which active tubular secretion is the major determinant of the renal excretory rate.

Some drugs are excreted (either unchanged but more usually as conjugates) in the bile. The unchanged drug or metabolite can then be reabsorbed directly although some conjugates are first metabolized by intestinal bacteria to the parent compound which is then reabsorbed. This can result in a prolongation of half-life and duration of action of the drug and probably occurs with warfarin and some antibiotics (e.g. erythromycin). The pathway may be particularly important in patients with reduced renal excretory capacity.

PHARMACODYNAMIC FACTORS

Drugs can produce a pharmacological action in four ways. They can: 1. interact with specific receptors; 2. inhibit physiological enzyme processes; 3. be incorporated into synthetic processes, or 4. act by a direct physical action.

1. An increasing number of specific receptors are being identified both on the cell surface and within the cell itself. These are specific sites which respond to very low concentrations of a so called 'agonist' to produce a characteristic biological response. To perform this function an agonist must firstly show an affinity for the receptor and secondly, be able to produce an effect. The latter ability is referred to as the drug's intrinsic activity. If the drug effect is plotted as a function of the logarithm of the drug concentration at the receptor site, it typically takes the shape shown in Fig. 2.2. Normally, however, the physician is using the drug in the central or loglinear portion of the dose response curve, since maximum effect may not be possible without unacceptable adverse effects. The affinity (and potency) of the drug is defined by the position of its log-dose response curve along the horizontal axis of the log-concentration response graph. The intrinsic activity (or efficacy) is defined as the maximum possible response (measured along the vertical axis).

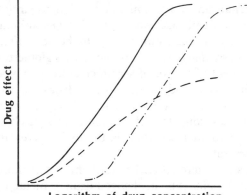

Fig. 2.2 Concentration response curves for: (a) an agonist drug (—); (b) the same agonist drug in the presence of a competitive antagonist (— . — . —) note the parallel shift to the right; (c) the agonist drug in the presence of a non-competitive antagonist (— — — —), note the non-parallel shift and the reduced maximum effect.

Some drugs may occupy the receptor site but have no intrinsic activity and therefore produce no response. Depending upon their concentration and affinity for the receptor relative to an agonist however, they can reduce the effect of the agonist and therefore are termed 'antagonists'. Full antagonists have no activity of their own, whereas partial agonists may behave as antagonists under certain circumstances. Competitive antagonists shift the dose-response curve of the agonist to the right in a parallel fashion. Other antagonists irreversibly bind to the receptor and reduce the intrinsic activity of the agonist (Fig. 2.2); the concentration response curve for these agonists will be shifted to the right but in a non-parallel fashion. It is by this mechanism that the alpha-adrenergic receptor antagonist, phenoxybenzamine, acts. The effect of phenoxybenzamine is prolonged because only when new receptor protein has been synthesized will this non-competitive antagonist's effects wear-off. There is evidence that the sensitivity of beta receptors to beta agonists and beta antagonists falls with age, although the mechanism is still unclear.

2. Some drugs act by inhibiting intracellular enzymic processes, either competitively or non-competitively. Methothrexate competes competitively with folinic acid for the enzyme dihydrofolate reductase, for example, whilst monoamineoxidase inhibitors (used in depression) appear to act irreversibly.

3. Other drugs are incorporated into biosynthetic products such as nucleoproteins. This is the mechanism of action of the purine analogues, azathiaprine and 6-mercaptopurine, which are used as cytotoxic agents. Metabolites of certain drugs (e.g. procainamide and paracetamol) may bind to DNA, and this may be the mechanism of their toxicity in certain individuals.

4. A number of agents act by physical action (e.g. osmotic, bulk and faecal softener purgatives). Local anaesthetics and general anaesthetics may also work in a similar fashion, since by diffusing into cell membranes they appear to discourage depolarization.

COMPLIANCE

Poor compliance is a major factor affecting drug response. It is particularly troublesome in the very young and the very old, patients with psychiatric disease, and those on long term therapy, especially when the disease produces few symptoms (e.g. hypertension). It may be suspected in patients who fail to respond to a reasonable dose of the drug and measurement of the drug concentration in plasma or urine may help to confirm this. It can only be diagnosed with certainty, however, if administration of the drug is supervised and subsequent plasma concentrations and/or biological effects are monitored.

Compliance can be improved in children by choosing medicines which are palatable. In all age groups it is improved by giving the drug in as few divided daily doses as possible, and keeping the number of drugs prescribed to any one patient to an absolute minimum. It is also important that the elderly and disabled be able to remove the drug from their container and in difficult cases, compliance aids such as small drug cabinets and calendar packs are available. A major factor in compliance is the doctor/patient relationship. If the doctor has the patient's conficence and has taken the time and trouble to explain the need for treatment and the possible adverse effects, the patient is much more likely to feel a participant in, rather than a passive recipient of, the therapeutic process.

FURTHER READING

Gibaldi M 1984 Biopharmaceutics and clinical pharmacokinetics. Lea and Febiger, Philadelphia

Smith S E, Rawlins M D (eds) 1973 Variability in human drug response. Butterworth, London

3

Adverse effects of drugs and therapeutic drug monitoring

Any substance which exerts useful therapeutic effects may also produce unwanted or adverse effects in some individuals. Indeed, adverse reaction to drugs are directly responsible for about 5% of hospital admissions. Even if admission was not precipitated by an adverse reaction, 10% of patients will develop an adverse effect to a drug while in hospital and 0.5% of patients who die in hospital do so as a direct result of their drug treatment rather than of the condition for which they were admitted.

The drugs most often involved are anticoagulants, antihypertensive agents and anti-rheumatic drugs, particularly the non-steroidal anti-inflammatory agents, although digoxin, corticosteroids and cytotoxic drugs are also often responsible. Adverse effects commonly involve the skin, central nervous system and the gastrointestinal tract. They are commoner at the extremes of life, (e.g. in neonates and the elderly) and women appear to be more at risk than men, although the reason for this is unknown. Patients with a history of allergy are prone to develop adverse reactions,

Table 3.1 Adverse effects related to hereditary enzyme deficiencies

Enzyme deficiency	Geographical features	Drugs involved	Adverse effects
Cholinesterase (serum or pseudocholinesterase)	World-wide	Succinylcholine	Prolonged neuromuscular blockade and apnoea
Glucose-6-phosphate dehydrogenase	Mediterranean and Negro races, Sephardic Jews	Primaquine Sulphonamides Nitrofurantoin Quinine Chloramphenicol Fava beans	Haemolysis
Erythrocyte diaphorase (methaemoglobin reductase)	World-wide	Sulphonamides Nitrites	Methaemoglobin-aemia

even if the reactions are not immunologically mediated; and someone who has already experienced an adverse reaction to a drug is more likely to experience a further reaction, even to a non-related drug. Patients with reduced ability to eliminate drug, either because of heart failure, liver disease or renal disease are also more at risk than other patients. Finally, there is evidence that racial and genetic factors may predispose to adverse reactions (see Table 3.1).

DOSE-DEPENDENT ADVERSE EFFECTS (Type A)

These have been termed Type A reactions because they are an 'accentuation' of the known pharmacological effect of the drug, whether this is the desired therapeutic effect or an undesired effect. Such reactions account for about three quarters of all adverse reactions and although they may cause considerable morbidity, are not generally associated with high mortality.

Dose-dependent adverse reactions may occur because of pharmaceutical characteristics of the drug, or pharmacokinetic or pharmacodynamic factors in a particular patient.

Pharmaceutical factors. A large proportion of many tablets consists of excipients (binding materials, dispersing agents and fillers). Changes in these materials can result in toxicity: a change in the method of formulation of digoxin resulted in an outbreak of dose-dependent toxicity, but recent more stringent regulatory controls have reduced the incidence of these problems.

Pharmacokinetic factors. Variability in all pharmacokinetic processes (absorption, distribution, metabolism and excretion) may be responsible for dose-dependent adverse effects in some patients given recommended doses of certain drugs. Examples of these types of reaction are given in Chapter 2.

Pharmacodynamic factors. Adverse reactions may occur due to abnormal response at the target organ. Thus hyperthyroid patients are more sensitive to the effect of digoxin and the elderly have a greater anticoagulant response than younger subjects to any given plama warfarin concentration and therefore require lower daily doses of the drug. Homeostatic mechanisms may be less adaptable in the elderly. This may be why they are more prone to drug-induced postural hypotension, and drug-related hypothermia.

DOSE-INDEPENDENT ADVERSE EFFECTS (Type B)

These have been termed, Type B, bizarre or idiosyncratic reactions. They are rarer than dose-dependent reactions and are less predictable, since the effects are apparently unrelated to the known pharmacology of the drug. Because of their lack of predictability, they have a higher mortality than Type A reactions. Their morbidity is low however if the patient survives the initial event.

Type B reactions can also occur due to pharmaceutical, pharmacokinetic or pharmacodynamic factors.

Pharmaceutical factors. Type B reactions may occur to inactive ingredients. Some preservatives, (e.g. chlorocresol or parabens), fillers such as lactose, (producing exacerbation of coeliac disease) and dyes (e.g. tartrazine) may cause Type B adverse reactions. Solubilising agents such as the ethylenediamine in aminophyline injection may also cause a dose independent allergic reaction which may be severe.

Pharmacokinetic factors. Some metabolites, although quantitatively unimportant, may result in toxicity. This may account for the hepatotoxicity due to isoniazid, but it is not clear why only some subjects should respond adversely.

Pharmacodynamic factors. Patients with hereditary enzyme deficiencies may be more prone to develop apparently dose-independent adverse effects. Haemolysis caused by dapsone and other oxidant drugs is commoner in patients with glucose 6-phosphate dehydrogenase (G 6PD) deficiency (Table 3.1). Similarly, some agents can cause intermittent porphyria in a dose-independent fashion (Table 3.2).

Table 3.2   Some drugs which may precipitate acute intermittent porphyria

1. Antibiotics	sulphonamides
	rifampicin
2. Anxiolytics	barbiturates
	chlordiazepoxide
	dichloralphenazone
	glutethimide
3. Alcohol	
4. Anticonvulsants	barbiturates
	phenytoin
	ethosuximide
5. Antihypertensives	methyldopa
6. Antidiabetics	tolbutamide
7. Antidepressants	imipramine
8. Antifungal agents	griseofulvin
9. Miscellaneous	ergotamine
	female sex hormones

DIAGNOSIS AND MANAGEMENT OF ADVERSE REACTIONS

The diagnosis of drug-induced disease can rarely be made with certainty. It has to be made by assessing the accumulation of evidence against an agent. The first priority is to take a full drug history, not only of all prescribed medicines, but also of 'over the counter' remedies, remembering that some patients do not consider the oral contraceptive as a drug, for example. It is also important to note the brand names of the agents being given, since different pharmaceutical formulations may result in a different spectrum of adverse effects. Because organs have a limited number of responses to noxious stimulae, physical examination rarely allows distinction between disease or drug-induced effects. Certain forms of skin discolouration, however (e.g. the blue discolouration associated with chlorpromazine or amiodarone) may point to a drug-induced effect and recurrence of an eczematous reaction at a fixed site on the body may indicate a fixed drug eruption. The usefulness of biochemical tests is similarly limited. Measurement of plasma drug concentrations may in some cases help to confirm the suspicion of dose dependent adverse effects. Measurement of acetylator status may also help, since it is extremely rare for example for drug-induced lupus erythematosus due to hydralazine to occur in a fast acetylator of the drug. The rate of resolution of symptoms in response to stopping the suspected drug is also of value in diagnosis. Rechallenge of the patient by administration of the drug topically, orally or systemically gives the strongest evidence of causation, but the risks of this procedure must be balanced against the potential benefit to the patient and it is therefore rarely performed.

PREVENTION OF ADVERSE REACTIONS

The risk of developing an adverse reaction increases disproportionately with the number of drugs prescribed. It is therefore important to review and rationalise drug therapy regularly. When a drug is prescribed, the prescription should be written legibly, preferably in block letters using the approved name. Illegible prescriptions have sometimes led to fatal adverse reactions. If an adverse reaction occurs, the patient's medical and prescription record should be identified with an eye-catching label indicating the reaction. Failure to do this has resulted in patients being re-exposed to drugs to which they have already had a severe reaction. Any severe adverse reaction to a drug should also be reported to the Committee of Safety of Medicines so that patterns of adverse effects can be studied nationally. Reports are made using a yellow card on which patient details and a list of the suspected drug and other drugs is reported. Any adverse reaction (no matter how minor) to a recently introduced drug (marked with an inverted black triangle in the British National Formulary) should also be reported. Only this approach has the potential power to detect reactions of low incidence.

In some clinical situations, the risk of an adverse reaction is such that certain drugs should be avoided if at all possible. Drugs to be avoided in pregnancy and during breast feeding are listed in Tables. 3.3 and 3.4.

Table 3.3 Drugs to avoid during pregnancy

1. Antibiotics	tetracycline
	trimethoprim
	aminoglycosides
	sulphonamides
2. Antithyroids	(and radioiodine)
3. Analgesics	opiates
	N.S.A.I.D.'s
4. Anticoagulants	(Oral)
5. Antineoplastics	
6. Antidiabetics	(Oral)
7. Androgens	progestogens and
	diethylstilboestrol
8. Miscellaneous	vitamin D
	vaccines (live)
	radioisotopes

Table 3.4 Drugs to avoid during breast feeding

1. Antibiotics	sulphonamides
	tetracyclines
	chloramphenicol
	isoniazid
2. Antithyroids	(and radioiodine)
3. Analgesics	opiates
4. Anticoagulants	phenindione
5. Antineoplastics	
6. Miscellaneous	lithium

THERAPEUTIC DRUG MONITORING

As has been mentioned earlier, monitoring of plasma drug concentration of certain drugs will help to reduce the incidence of adverse effects as well as to improve drug efficacy and detect non-compliance. It is necessary first to discuss some pharmacokinetic concepts before describing when and how to take samples for drug analysis.

When a drug is given intravenously its concentration generally falls in an exponential fashion. In the simplest situation (e.g. after warfarin) the drug falls monoexponentially but the decline of some other drugs can follow a bi- or triexponential pattern. The time taken for the drug concentration to fall from any value to half of that value will be constant under 'first-order' conditions. This time is referred to as the elimination half-life or $T\frac{1}{2}$ (Fig. 3.1). If the drug concentration is expressed on a logarithmic scale the exponential curve becomes a straight line (Fig. 2.1 p. 20) and the intercept of this line on the y axis after intravenous administration is known as C_0 the theoretical concentration immediately after drug administration. The apparent distribution volume of the drug (Vd) is calculated by dividing the dose of drug given by the concentration, C_0. Drug clearance, the volume of plasma completely cleared of drug per unit time, can be calculated using the following equation:

(1) Clearance $= Vd \times 0.693/T\frac{1}{2}$

or (2) Clearance $=$ Dose/AUC
where AUC is the area under the plasma concentration time curve from time zero to infinity (Fig. 3.1).

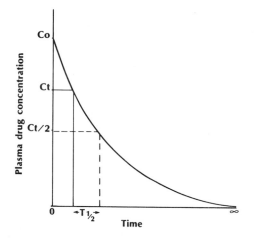

Fig. 3.1 Relationship between plasma drug concentration and time after intravenous administration for a drug undergoing first order elimination with a mono-exponential pattern.

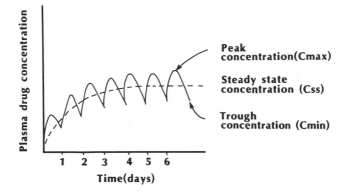

Fig. 3.2 Time course of plasma drug concentration after repeated daily oral administration of a drug with $T_{\frac{1}{2}}$ of 24 hrs.

The value for drug clearance is expressed in units of volume per unit time (e.g. litres per minute). It is the sum of all the clearance by all the organs of elimination, thus total plasma clearance is equal to renal clearance plus metabolic clearance of drug.

After oral administration, an initial absorption phase is seen before the drug is eliminated in a similar fashion as after intravenous administration (Fig. 2.1 page 20). The average drug concentration after repeated doses will continue to rise, until steady state condition is reached when the amount of drug eliminated from the body is equal to the dose administered (Fig. 3.2). The full effect of a drug will therefore not be felt until at least five half-lives have elapsed. The steady state concentration (Css) is an average drug concentration during the dosing interval at steady state, determined by the following equation:

(3) $Css = Dose \times F/Clearance \times \tau$

Where τ (tau) is the time interval between doses and F is the fraction of the administered dose which reaches the systemic circulation without being metabolized (bioavailability). Bioavailability can be calculated by dividing the area under the curve after oral administration by the area under the curve after intravenous administration of the same dose of drug. Bioavailability may be less than unity, either if the drug is not completely absorbed from the gastrointestinal tract (e.g. cimetidine) or if the drug is metabolized either in the gut (e.g. isoprenaline), the liver (e.g. propranolol) or the lung (e.g. noradrenaline). It readily becomes apparent from this equation that if the total dose of drug given per day remains the same the average steady state concentration (Css) during the day will be unchanged, although if larger doses are given at more infrequent intervals the difference between the peak and trough concentration will increase (Fig. 3.2). This will of course be important if the adverse effects of the drug are related to its peak concentration or if there is a threshold concentration below which drug effect is not obtained. The longer the half-life of the drug, the longer can the interval between doses be for any given difference between peak and trough concentration. Equation 3 also illustrates that the steady state concentration will be directly proportional to the daily dose, provided that bioavailability remains constant. While this is true for most drugs, some compounds (e.g. ethanol and phenytoin) have saturable hepatic metabolic routes so that the clearance falls with increasing dose. A small increase in dose may then produce a disproportionately large increase in the steady state concentration so that proportionality does not apply.

From the previous considerations it is apparent that at least four and preferably five half-lives should normally elapse between starting the drug or changing its dosage before sampling to enable steady state to be reached. However if it is suspected that toxic effects may occur or have occurred due to excessive accumulation of the drug, earlier sampling might be helpful. Since the rate of drug absorption may vary due to several factors outlined in the last chapter, a trough level taken just before the next dose is normally best related to the steady state concentration. If peak levels are important, samples should be taken two to three hours after an oral dose or later if a sustained release formula has been given. For the aminoglycosides, blood should be taken just before the next dose for the trough concentration, and a half to one hour after an intravenous injection or one hour after an intramuscular injection. For digoxin it is preferable to wait at least 8 hours after administration of an oral dose before sampling and for lithium it is conventional to draw the sample in the morning, 12 hours after the evening dose. In patients receiving intravenous infusions, it is normally necessary to wait at least 2 to 4 hours after the last change in the infusion rate before sampling. Details of sampling time relative to the last dose should always be put on the drug assay request form.

The total drug concentration may not, in certain circumstances, mirror the free drug concentration (e.g. in liver and renal disease) and for some drugs salivary concentrations may provide a closer approximation to the latter. Monitoring of saliva concentration is

Table 3.5 Drugs for which plasma concentration monitoring is useful

Drug	Usual half-life (hours)	Usual therapeutic plasma concentration	Toxic levels	Elimination	Special risks
Amikacin	2	trough < 10 mg/l peak 20–30 mg/l	trough > 10 mg/l peak > 40 mg/l	R	RD, E
Carbamazepine	15–30	plasma 21–42 umol/l saliva 4.0–10.5 umol/l	> 42 μmol/l > 10.5 μmol/l	M	LD
Digoxin	30–40	1.3–2.6 nmol/l	> 2.6 nmol/l	R	RD, E
Digitoxin	120–168	13–45 nmol/l	> 45 nmol/l	M	LD
Disopyramide	4–8	9–18 μmol/l	> 24 μmol/l	M/R	RD
Gentamicin	2	trough < 2 mg/l peak 4–8 mg/l	trough > 2 mg/l peak > 12 mg/l	R	RD, E
Lignocaine	2–4	9.0–22.0 μmol/l	> 22.0 μmol/l	M	LD, CF
Lithium	7–20	0.6–1.4 mmol/l	> 1.5 mmol/l	R	RD
Mexiletine	4–8	5.5–11 μmol/l	> 16.5 μmol/l	M/R	RD, LD
Netilmicin	2	trough < 3 mg/l peak 6–10 mg/l	trough > 4 mg/l peak > 12 mg/l	R	RD, E
Phenobarbitone	60–160	65–170 μmol/l	> 170 μmol/l	R	RD, E
Phenytoin	20–60	plasma 40–80 μmol/l (i) saliva 4–8 μmol/l	> 80 μmol/l > 8 μmol/l	M	LD, RD
Salicylate	8–24	1–2.1 μmol/l (i)	>2.9 μmol/l	M/R	LD, RD
Sodium valproate	6–12	350–700 μmol	?	M	LD,
Theophylline	8–20	plasma 55–110 μmol/l saliva 40–80 μmol/l	plasma > 110 μmol/l	M	LD, CF
Tobramycin	2	trough < 2 mg/l peak 4–8 mg/l	trough > 2 mg/l peak > 12 mg/l	R	RD, E

Note: Therapeutic range needs to be decreased for low albumin concentration and/or renal failure R = renal M = metabolism RD = renal disease LD = liver disease E = elderly patients CF = cardiac failure also preferable if possible in young children in order to avoid venepuncture. Saliva flow can be stimulated by using two drops of citric acid on the tongue and saliva may be useful particularly for measurement of phenytoin and theophylline concentrations. Acetylator phenotype can be determined by measurement of plasma drug concentrations after administration of izoniazid, dapsone or sulphadimidine. The generally accepted therapeutic ranges for the commonly measured drugs are shown in Table 3.5.

FURTHER READING

Davies D M 1977 Textbook of adverse drug reactions, Oxford University Press
Richens A, Marks V (eds) 1981 Therapeutic drug monitoring. Churchill
    Livingstone, Edinburgh

4

Mechanisms of drug interaction

It is common for patients to be treated with more than one drug at the same time, and there are several different ways in which they may interact for the patient's good or harm. The following is a general summary of some of the principal mechanisms involved.

PHARMACOKINETIC INTERACTIONS

1. Formulation incompatibility

Drugs may interact with so-called 'inert' constituents of the formulations in which they are compounded, and this may influence their biological availability (see pp. 5 and 12). This applies equally to oral and parenteral preparations.

2. Absorption

Drugs which influence the rate of gastric emptying may modify the rate of absorption of other drugs (see p. 184). Chelation or other forms of binding of drugs within the gastrointestinal tract may reduce their absorption. Ferrous compounds and calcium, magnesium and aluminium-containing antacids chelate with tetracyclines to reduce the absorption of the latter. The anion-exchange resin cholestyramine can reduce the absorption of digoxin, thiazide diuretics, thyroxine and paracetamol.

Vasoconstrictor drugs are combined with local anaesthetic agents in some parenteral formulations to restrict their area of action at the injection site.

3. Protein binding (see p. 16)

4. Enzyme induction (see p. 18)

5. Enzyme inhibition

35

Some drugs, such as sulthiame and cimetidine, may inhibit drug metabolizing enzymes and so prolong the plasma half-lives of some other drugs. Treatment with monoamine oxidase inhibitors leads to accumulation of monoamines such as adrenaline, noradrenaline, dopamine and 5-hydroxytryptamine within the central and autonomic nervous systems, and also prevents the hepatic metabolism of other exogenous monoamines such as tyramine. This is the basis of their important interactions with certain drugs and foodstuffs (see p. 39).

Organo-phosphorus anticholinesterases instilled into the conjunctival sac in the treatment of glaucoma may be absorbed sufficiently to produce resistance to neuro-muscular blockade by tubocurarine.

Enzyme inhibition is also the basis of action of many chemotherapeutic agents used in treatment of infectious and neoplastic conditions. Synergism between drugs may occur if they act on different enzyme systems within the cells of an infecting organism or in a neoplastic cell. For example, in the combination product cotrimoxazole, sulphamethoxazole inhibits the conversion of para-aminobenzoic acid to folic acid, and trimethoprim inhibits the conversion of folic acid to folinic acid, sequential steps in the same metabolic pathway (see Ch. 19).

6. Excretion (see p. 20)

PHARMACODYNAMIC INTERACTIONS

1. Electrolyte changes

Drug-induced changes in electrolyte concentrations may influence the action of some other drugs. The best example of such an interaction is the potentiation of action of digitalis glycosides by diuretic-induced hypokalaemia.

2. Blockade of neuronal uptake

An important mechanism in the termination of action of noradrenaline is its active reuptake into noradrenergic neurones. Blockade of this reuptake process poteniates the pressor action of noradrenaline and adrenaline and of other substances that also depend on the same uptake process, such as phenylephrine. Among the groups of drugs which may block neuronal uptake are the tricyclic antidepressants (e.g. imipramine) and some adrenergic neurone blocking drugs (e.g. guanethidine, bethanidine).

Some indirectly acting sympathomimetic amines (e.g. tyramine) and some adrenergic neurone blocking drugs (e.g. guanethidine, bethanidine) depend for their pharmacological effects on being taken up into the neurone through the same uptake process as noradrenaline. Their action may, therefore, be prevented or reversed, by treatment with tricyclic antidepressant drugs.

3. Transmitter depletion

The effects of drugs which depend for their action on release of neurotransmitter substances may be reduced by the administration of other drugs which produce neurotransmitter depletion. For example, pressor responses to tyramine are reduced in reserpinised subjects.

4. Receptor blockade

The development of selective receptor blocking drugs, particularly in the autonomic nervous system and its effector organs, has led to several important clinical interactions. For example, a-adrenergic receptor blockade prevents the pressor effects of sympathomimetic amines, and β-receptor blockade reduces or abolishes their cardiac stimulating activity. Similarly, the anti-cholinergic action of several different classes of drugs (e.g. tricyclic antidepressants, antihistamines) reduces the effects of cholinomimetic agents.

FUNCTIONAL SUMMATION OF EFFECTS

Drugs which produce a pharmacological effect by different biochemical mechanisms may have a synergistic interaction, for example, the mutual enhancement of the central nervous system depressant activity of anaesthetics, hypnotics, sedatives, tranquillizers and narcotic analgesics.

Other examples include the potentiation of the action of oracl anticoagulant drugs by broad spectrum antibiotics which reduce vitamin K absorption, and by aspirin which inhibits prothrombin synthesis, as well as competing for plasma protein binding sites.

Catecholamines normally elevate the blood sugar level, and blockade of this effect by propranolol will potentiate the effect of oral hypoglycaemic agents.

Table 4.1 Some clinically important drug interactions and their underlying mechanisms when known

Drug A may interact with	Drug B	Potential results	Mechanism
Reduced absorption			
Tetracyclines	Antacids Oral iron Oral zinc	Reduced absorption of A	Chelation
Hepatic enzyme induction			
Barbiturates	Coumarin anticoagulants	Reduced activity of B	Hepatic enzyme induction by A
Phenytoin	Corticosteroids	Reduced activity of B	
Carbamazepine	Oral contraceptives	Contraceptive failure	
Rifampicin	Sodium valproate	Reduced plasma levels of B	
Reduced hepatic extraction			
Carbamazepine	Cimetidine	Potentiation of A	
Phenytoin			
Diazepam			
Propranolol			
Theophylline	Sodium valproate	Potentiation of A	
Carbamazepine	Chloramphenicol		
Coumarin anticoagulants	Cimetidine Phenylbutazone Sulphonamides Tolbutamide Indomethacin Phenytoin Clofibrate	Potentiation of A	Displacement of A by B from plasma protein binding sites may produce transient potentiation as an additional mechanism of potentiation.

Drug A	Drug B	Effect	Mechanism
Reduced renal excretion			
Penicillins Cephalosporins Dapsone Mexiletine	Probenecid	Increased plasma levels of A	Reduced tubular secretion of A
	Antacids	Increased plasma levels of A	Reduced excretion in alkaline urine
Inhibition of neuronal uptake			
Monoamine reuptake inhibiting antidepressants e.g. imipramine amitriptyline Mazindol	Bethanidine Debrisoquine Guanethidine	Reduction of antihypertensive action of B	Inhibition by A of neuronal uptake of B
	Noradrenaline Adrenaline Phenylephrine	Potentiation of pressor action of B	Inhibition by A of neuronal uptake of B
Inhibition of monoamine oxidase			
Monoamine oxidase inhibitors e.g. phenelzine	Indirectly-acting sympathomimetics Fenfluramine Levodopa Tyramine-containing foods and wines	Acute adrenergic hypertensive crisis	Release by B of monoamine stores, increased by A
	Pethidine and other narcotics	Central nervous excitation, coma	Uncertain but may involve increased 5HT activity

Table 4.1 Some clinically important drug interactions and their underlying mechanisms when known

Drug A may interact with	Drug B	Potential results	Mechanism
Summation of effects			
Barbiturates	Alcohol	Increased CNS depression	
Benzodiazepines	Other CNS depressants		
Monoamine reuptake inhibiting undepressants e.g. imipramine amitriptyline	Anticholinergics Antihistamines	Excessive central and peripheral atropine-like effects	Summation of anticholinergic effects
	Antiparkinsonian drugs Antipsychotic drugs		
	Monoamine oxidase inhibitors, e.g. phenelzine	Central nervous excitation, hyperpyrexia, coma	Increased central monoamine activity
Thiazide and loop diuretics	Corticosteroids Carbenoxolone	Hypokalaemia	Increased urinary potassium loss
Captopril	Potassium-sparing diuretics	Hyperkalaemia	Potassium retention
Antiarrhythmic drugs	Beta-adrenoceptor blockers, particularly propranolol	Myocardial depression Hypotension	
Antihypertensive drugs	Vasodilators Alcohol Fenfluramine Levodopa Bromocriptine	Hypotension	
Aminoglycosides e.g. gentamicin	Loop diuretics	Increased nephrotoxicity Increased ototoxicity	
Cephaloridine Cephalothin			

Others

Drug A	Drug B	Effect	Mechanism
Digoxin	Thiazides and loop diuretics	Digitalis toxicity	Hypokalaemia
Digoxin	Quinidine, amiodarone nifedipine, verapamil	Increased digoxin plasma levels, risk of toxicity	Reduced digoxin clearance
Thiazides and loop diuretics	Non-steroidal anti-inflammatory drugs	Reduced diuretic and antihypertensive effect of A	May involve inhibition of prostaglandin synthesis
Beta-adrenoceptor blocking drugs	Non-steroidal anti-inflammatory drugs	Reduced antihypertensive effect of A	May involve inhibition of prostaglandin synthesis
Lithium	Diuretics	Lithium retention and toxicity	Lithium retained as sodium excreted
Lithium	Haloperidol	Increased incidence of extrapyramidal effects	Uncertain
Competitive neuromuscular blocking drugs, e.g. tubocurare	Aminoglycosides Propranolol Lithium Quinidine	Potentiated neuromuscular blockade	Uncertain
Metronidazole Chlorpropamide Alcohol	Alcohol	Facial flushing	Uncertain
Alcohol	Disulfiram	Antabuse' reaction: facial flushing, tachycardia hypotension, arrhythmias	Inhibition by B of metabolism of A to produce acetaldehyde accumulation
Theophylline	Erythromycin	Increased plasma level of A, decrease of B	May involve inhibition of hepatic metabolism of A by B, and increased clearance of B by A
Azathioprine 6-Mercaptopurine	Allopurinol	Increased toxicity of A	Xanthine-oxidase inhibition by B

The action of antihypertensive drugs may be increased by compounds such as alcohol which possess a general vasodilating action. On the other hand, their effects may be reduced by corticosteroids and non-steroidal anti-inflammatory drugs. Sodium retention may account for this interaction, but inhibition of prostaglandin synthesis may also be involved (page 219).

Clinically important drug interactions

A large number of drug interactions have been demonstrated in clinical studies, in normal human volunteers or in vitro systems, but not all are of clinical importance. Some examples of interactions of potential clinical importance are given in Table 4.1 with their underlying mechanisms when known.

SUGGESTIONS FOR FURTHER READING

Davies D M 1981 Textbook of adverse drug reactions, 2nd edn. Oxford University Press
Stockley I 1981 Drug interactions. Blackwell, Oxford

5

Autonomic drugs

AUTONOMIC GANGLIA

Stimulation of preganglionic nerve fibres to autonomic ganglia, both sympathetic and parasympathetic, results in the liberation of acetylcholine. Injection of very small amounts of acetylcholine into the perfusion fluid of an isolated ganglion, or into the blood supply of a ganglion produces excitation of the ganglion cells. Acetylcholinesterase is also present in the ganglia to inactivate rapidly the acetylcholine after release and receptor stimulation. This is good evidence that acetylcholine is the physiological neurotransmitter in autonomic ganglia.

The ganglionic actions of acetylcholine are referred to as its nicotinic actions, because nicotine has similar effects on autonomic ganglia. There is initial stimulation and then blockade of the ganglion cells. The effects may be summarized as:

Cardiovasular system — stimulation of sympathetic ganglia and the adrenal medulla results in release of catecholamines producing vasoconstriction, tachycardia and elevated blood pressure.

Gastrointestinal tract — initially there is increased tone and peristalsis due to parasympathetic stimulation. With higher concentrations of acetylcholine autonomic blockade occurs, with reduction of intestinal tone and motility.

Glandular secretions — initial stimulation of salivary and bronchial secretions is followed by inhibition.

Drugs blocking autonomic ganglia

It is possible to classify drugs blocking autonomic ganglia according to their mechanism of action:

(a) Depolarizing drugs, which produce a state of prolonged depolarization of the ganglion cell membrane so that the neurotransmitter cannot generate activity in the cell. Nicotine is an example of such a compound. Although of considerable pharmacological interest, depolarizing drugs have little therapeutic value as they have an initial ganglion-stimulating effect before producing blockade.

(b) Competitive blocking drugs, where the drug competes with acetylcholine for receptor sites on the ganglion cell membrane. These drugs can be further subdivided on a chemical basis:

(i) quaternary ammonium compounds, e.g. hexamethonium, pentolinium

(ii) secondary amines, e.g. mecamylamine

(iii) tertiary amines, e.g. pempidine.

Although the quaternary ammonium compounds are potent ganglion blocking agents, they are highly ionized and therefore poorly absorbed through the gastrointestinal mucous membrane. They are, therefore, unsuitable for oral administration and must be given parenterally for predictable therapeutic efficacy. Secondary amines such as mecamylamine are somewhat better absorbed, and tertiary amines, such as pempidine, are sufficiently unionized at gut pH for satisfactory blood levels to be achieved by oral administration.

Effect of autonomic ganglion blockade

Cardiovascular system — ganglionic blockade produces vasodilatation, peripheral pooling of blood, decreased venous return and cardiac output, and hypotension. Under resting conditions the heart is under parasympathetic inhibitory control and blockade therefore results in tachycardia.

Gastrointestinal and urinary tracts — reduction in tone and motility produce constipation in the gut and urinary retention in the bladder.

Glandular secretions — dry mouth (xerostomia) and loss of sweating (anhidrosis) occur.

Eye — pupil dilation (mydriasis) and paralysis of accommodation.

Genital system — impotence may occur.

PERIPHERAL CHOLINERGIC NERVE TERMINAL

The actions of acetylcholine at the peripheral autonomic cholinergic nerve ending are known as its muscarinic actions, because they are mimicked by muscarine, an alkaloid derived from various species of mushroom. They may be summarized as follows:

Cardiovascular system — vasodilatation and marked slowing of the heart producing a fall in blood pressure.

Gastrointestinal tract — smooth muscles are stimulated, increasing tone and motility, with higher concentrations of acetylcholine causing spasm and tenesmus. The tone and motility of the gall bladder and bile ducts are also increased.

Glandular secretions — salivary, lachrymal, gastric, pancreatic, intestinal and mucous cells generally are stimulated.

Urogenital and respiratory tracts — smooth muscle in the bronchi, ureters and urinary bladder is stimulated leading to broncho-spasm and voiding of urine.

Eye — there is pupillary constriction, spasm of accommodation and a transitory rise in intraocular pressure followed by a more persistent fall.

Cholinomimetic drugs

Drugs mimicking the actions of acetylcholine may be divided into:

(a) Derivatives of acetylcholine e.g. methacholine, carbachol, bethanechol.

(b) Other alkaloids, e.g. pilocarpine, muscarine, arecoline.

(c) Anticholinesterase drugs which inhibit or inactivate acetylcholinesterase and so allow acetylcholine to accumulate at cholinergic receptor sites and produce its effects. The most important of these in clinical practice are neostigmine, physostigmine, pyridostigmine, edrophonium, ambenonium and distigmine.

Drugs blocking the peripheral autonomic cholinergic junction

Parasympathetic effector organs vary in their sensitivity to the blocking effect of drugs. The most sensitive are salivary, bronchial and sweat glands which are inhibited by small concentrations. Larger doses dilate the pupils, paralyse accommodation of the eye, and block vagal tone on the heart. Still larger doses inhibit parasympathetic control of the bladder and gastrointestinal tract. Gastric secretion is the most resistant to blockade. Most drugs which block the peripheral cholinergic junction act by competitive inhibition of acetylcholine at the receptor site. This means that their action can be overcome by increasing the concentration of transmitter at the receptor site, for example by administration of an anticholinesterase drug which prevents its breakdown and allows it to accumulate until it has overcome the block.

Atropine and hyoscine

These are alkaloids derived from the belladonna plants and have been used as poisons and for medicinal purposes for thousands of years. Atropine is the racemic mixture of equal parts of D- and L-hyoscyamine, most of the antimuscarinic action residing in the L-isomer, L-Hyoscine (scopolamine) is the active isomer, the D-isomer having no clinical importance.

The effects of atropine and hyoscine are as follows:

Eye — pupil dilatation (mydriasis) due to blockade of cholinergic tone on the sphincter pupillae. The ciliary muscle of the lens is also paralysed producing impairment of accommodation (cycloplegia), the lens being fixed for far vision. Normal pupillary reflex constriction to light or convergence is abolished. Pupil dilatation may lead to a reduction in aqueous outflow and a rise in intraocular pressure in glaucomatous patients.

Cardiovascular system — small doses of atropine slow the heart but larger doses progressively block the vagus until at a dose of about 0.04 mg/kg body weight, vagal tone is completely removed and there is a tachycardia. During the initial slowing of heart there may be disturbances of atrioventricular conduction with electrocardiographic changes.

Gastrointestinal tract — salivary secretions are inhibited producing dryness of the mouth and difficulty in talking and swallowing. There is a reduction in gut motility, and there may be associated retention of urine.

Respiratory tract — inhibition of secretion in the nose, mouth, pharynx and bronchi leads to drying of the respiratory mucous membranes. This is accompanied by a reduction in airways resistance and increase in volume of residual air.

Central nervous system — atropine and hyoscine differ in their effects on the central nervous system. Atropine stimulates the medulla and cerebral cortex leading first to increased vagal tone and respiratory activity, in higher doses to excitation, restlessness, hallucinations and delirium, and finally to medullary paralysis and death. Hyoscine, on the other hand, usually causes drowsiness and euphoria, although occasionally it may cause atropine-like excitation. It has a depressant action on vestibular function and is useful in the management of motion sickness. Both drugs have anti-tremor activity which is the basis of their use in the treatment of Parkinson's disease.

Drugs with atropine-like activity

For gastrointestinal disturbances — propantheline bromide and poldine methylsulphate reduce gastric acid secretion and are used in management of peptic ulceration. Atropine methylnitrate is used in the medical treatment of congenital hypertrophic pyloric stenosis in infants. Dicyclomine is used in gastrointestinal colicky conditions particularly in infants. Other atropine-like drugs used as gut spasmolytics include glycopyrronium, mepenzolate, penthienate, pipenzolate, piperidolate and clidinium.

Mydriatics — the mydriatic effect of atropine eye drops lasts for a week or more. Homatropine hydrobromide has a more rapid action which is over in 48 hours. Eucatropine hydrochloride is another short-acting alternative with little, if any, effect on accommodation. Tropicamide with a duration of action of 3 hours, lachesine, about 6 hours, and cyclopentolate, about 24 hours, are widely used as mydriatic and cycloplegic agents.

Some monoamine reuptake inhibiting antidepressives — such as amitriptyline — see Chapter 7.

Antiparkinsonian drugs — see Chapter 6.

ADRENERGIC NERVE ENDING

Light and electron microscopical techniques show that sympathetic nerves end in terminal ramifications which have a beaded appearance, and fluorescent studies show that these varicosities contain granules of noradrenaline. The steps in the synthesis of noradrenaline and adrenaline are:

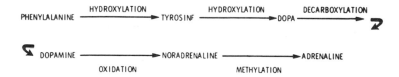

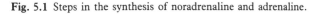

Fig. 5.1 Steps in the synthesis of noradrenaline and adrenaline.

Each step is controlled by enzymatic activity, but none of the enzymes is specific to adrenaline synthesis, and each takes part in other pathways. For example, L-aromatic amino acid decarboxylase, or dopa decarboxylase, also produces 5-hydroxytryptamine and histamine from their corresponding amino acids. The rate limiting step in this pathway is the conversion of tyrosine to dopa under the influence of tyrosine hydroxylase, and it may be blocked by certain drugs such as α-methyl paratyrosine.

Noradrenaline is found in the adrenal medulla and in the post-ganglionic sympathetic fibres. It disappears within a few days after never section. Adrenaline also is found in the adrenal medulla and in chromaffin cells elsewhere, but only insignificant amounts are found in sympathetic nerves.

It is probable that noradrenaline in sympathetic nerve terminals is in several stores or pools (Fig. 5.2). About 40% is in the cytoplasm and the other 60% is in granular stores or vesicles where it is bound to protein. It diffuses freely and passively from the granules into the cytoplasm and from the cytoplasm through the neuronal cell membrane into the extracellular space. It is carried in the opposite direction by active transport mechanisms from the extracellular space into the cytoplasm, and from the cytoplasm into

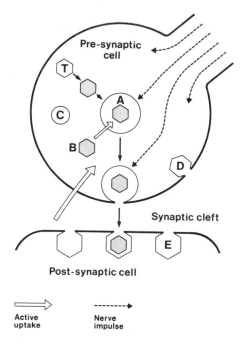

Fig. 5.2 Diagrammatic representation of adrenergic nerve ending and receptor. A, granular pool of noradrenaline; B, cytoplasmic pool of noradrenaline; C, monoamine oxidase; D, presynaptic receptor; E, postsynaptic receptor; T, precursor of noradrenaline (tyrosine, etc).

the granules. Binding of noradrenaline to protein within the granules probably represents a separate active process.

The noradrenaline in sympathetic nerve endings is, therefore, derived from two sources:

1. Local synthesis from phenylalanine.

2. Uptake from the extracellular space of noradrenaline, released locally, from distant sites such as the adrenal medulla, or exogenously administered. An understanding of this uptake process is important from the point of view of inactivation of noradrenaline after it has acted at the receptor site, for its granular binding represents a way in which it can be inactivated but used again. It seems likely, in fact, that uptake and storage represent its major route of inactivation under normal conditions, and that enzymatic breakdown plays only a minor role. For this reason the excretion rates of urinary metabolites of noradrenaline bear little relationship to adrenergic function under normal conditions. Uptake and storage of noradrenaline are also important because they represent possible sites of action of drugs which influence adrenergic activity.

The enzymatic breakdown of noradrenaline and adrenaline is largely dependent on two enzymes, monoamine oxidase (MAO) and catechol-O-methyltransferase (COMT). MAO is widely distributed throughout the body and is concerned with the intracellular metabolism of adrenaline, noradrenaline, dopamine and 5-hydroxytryptamine. COMT is responsible for the extraneuronal metabolism of noradrenaline and adrenaline which has been released from the adrenal medulla or from sympathetic nerves.

The mechanism by which the sympathetic nerve impulse releases noradrenaline from the nerve ending is not yet known in detail. In the adrenal medulla acetylcholine is liberated by preganglionic fibres and its interaction with receptors on the chromaffin cells results in release of adrenaline and noradrenaline. An intermediate step involves the entrance of calcium ions into the cells.

It is probable that the noradrenaline released by nerve impulses is that fraction in the granular or vesicular form. If so, then the release of noradrenaline from the sympathetic nerve may involve mechanisms similar to those releasing catecholamines from the adrenal medulla and chromaffin tissue elsewhere, and those releasing secretions from other cells throughout the body including insulin from the pancreas, histamine from mast cells and enzymes from digestive glands. In each case the secretion is stored in vesicles similar to those of noradrenaline in the adrenergic neurone.

Theory of stimulus secretion coupling

The theory runs as follows: the secretory product, in this case noradrenaline, is stored in subcellular granules enveloped by a membrane. Release of the substance depends on a process of exocytosis in which the full granule moves towards the periphery of the cell until the granular membrane fuses with the cell membrane under the influence of calcium ions. The cell-granular membrane then ruptures and the contents of the granule are released from the cell. The granular membrane then separates from the cell membrane and is retained for further use. The stimulus to this process varies from one type of cell to another. In the case of the neurone it is a nerve impulse, but the mechanism by which it triggers the process of exocytosis is unknown.

Presynaptic inhibition of facilitation

As well as stimulating receptors on the postsynaptic cell membrane, noradrenaline stimulates receptors on the presynaptic membrane (Fig. 5.3) and this acts, through a feedback mechanism, to regulate its further release. Similar mechanisms probably operate in other

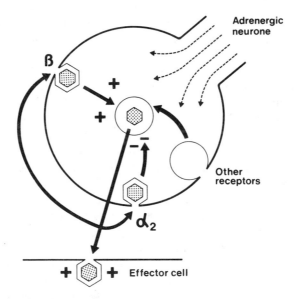

Fig. 5.3 Diagrammatic representation of adrenergic nerve ending and presynaptic and postsynaptic receptors. Presynaptic receptors may facilitate (β) or inhibit (α2) transmitter release (see p. 53).

systems, including dopaminergic and 5-hydroxytryptaminergic neurones. Blockade of these receptors can lead either to inhibition or facilitation of transmitter release (see p. 53).

SYMPATHOMIMETIC AMINES

Sympathomimetic amines, which resemble sympathetic nerve stimulation in their effects, may be divided into three groups on the basis of their mode of action.

(a) *Directly acting amines*. These have a direct action on sympathetic effector cells interacting with receptor sites on the cell membrane. They are, therefore, effective when the sympathetic nerve is depleted of its noradrenaline stores, either pharmacologically, or following sympathetic denervation. In fact, their action may be increased by such procedures to produce the phenomenon of 'denervation supersensitivity'. At least two factors seem to contribute to denervation supersensitivity. Firstly, there is a lack of the normal uptake process into the neurone, thus increasing amine concentration at the receptor site. Secondly, there appears to be an increase in the number of receptor sites, a response, presumably, of the postsynaptic cell to reduced transmitter stimulation. This increase is called 'up-regulation' while a reduction in receptor sites following sustained increase in synaptic transmitter concentrations is called 'down regulation'. Most of the directly acting amines are derivatives of catechol and so are called catecholamines. They include adrenaline, noradrenaline, isoprenaline and dopamine. Phenylephrine is a directly acting amine which is not a catecholamine.

(b) *Indirectly acting amines*. These compounds, most of them non-catecholamines, act by being taken up into the adrenergic nerve ending and releasing noradrenaline on to the receptor site. Their action is reduced or abolished, therefore, by surgical or pharmacological denervation which depletes the neuronal noradrenaline content. Examples of this type are tyramine, phenylpropanolamine, amphetamine and pseudoephedrine.

(c) *Mixed action amines*. Some amines such as ephedrine and methoxamine have both direct and indirect actions, which vary according to the species and tissue being studied.

ADRENERGIC RECEPTORS

Neurohumoral agents and transmitters such as acetylcholine and noradrenaline-like drugs, are composed of molecules. The result of their action on effector cells must be explained in terms of an interaction of these molecules, or parts of them, with specific molecules in the effector cell. The latter are called the 'specific receptors' for the transmitter or drug with respect to the particular effect. Other drug — tissue interactions that do not initiate such specific effects, such as binding of drugs to plasma proteins, binding of neurotransmitter to cell protein, and binding to enzymes for transport, storage and biotransformation are referred to in other terms such as 'secondary receptors', 'storage sites' or 'drug acceptors'.

In 1948, Ahlquist suggested that the effects of adrenaline at peripheral sympathetic sites could be divided into two groups with two types of postsynaptic receptor, α and β. These were originally called excitatory and inhibitory receptors, respectively, because of their general tendency to produce excitation or inhibition when

Table 5.1 Drugs which stimulate or block postganglionic sympathetic receptors

Receptor	Selectively activated by	Selectively blocked by		Main actions of receptor stimulation
α	Noradrenaline Phenylephrine Methoxamine	Phenoxybenz-amine Phentolamine Thymoxamine Indoramin Prazosin		Vasoconstriction of skin, splanchnic and coronary vessels Pupil dilatation Relaxation of gut Bronchoconstriction Hyperglycaemia and increase in plasma FFA
β_1	Dobutamine	Alprenolol Nadolol Oxprenolol Pindolol Propranolol Sotalol Timolol	Acebutolol Atenolol Betaxolol Metoprolol Practolol	Increased inotropic and chronotropic cardiac action
β_2	Fenoterol Isoetharine Orciprenaline Reproterol Rimiterol Salbutamol Terbutaline			Vasodilatation of coronary skeletal muscle and some skin vessels

Bronchial relaxation Tremor Relaxation of uterus Hyperglycaemia and increase in plasma FFA* |

* It is uncertain, at present, in which of the β-receptor subdivisions these actions should be included. Adrenaline activates both α-receptors and β-receptors. Labetalol blocks both α and β receptors.

stimulated, but as there are important exceptions to this in both groups it is proposed to refer to them as α or β-receptors. The β-group were then subdivided into β_1 and β_2-receptors. Important receptor actions and examples of compounds which selectively activate or block these receptors are given in Table 5.1. Adrenaline has both α and β actions and its effects will be the result of summation of these actions when they are interrelated.

Presynaptic receptors (see p. 50) appear to be of both α- and β-type; the latter possess a low threshold for stimulation and cause facilitation of noradrenaline release, while the α-receptors have a higher threshold and inhibit release. This may be seen as a regulatory mechanism, at first amplifying the transmitter action and then reducing or even terminating it. Presynaptic α-receptor blockade will, of course, facilitate transmitter release while β-blockade will inhibit it. By convention postsynaptic α receptors are called α_1 and presynaptic receptors α_2, but this is probably an oversimplification, receptors with α_2 pharmacological properties having been demonstrated on the postsynaptic membrane in some experimental preparations. It should be noted that this method of classification does not apply to β-receptors, although it appears that presynaptic β-receptors have the pharmacological properties of β_2 receptors.

It is probable that the adrenergic receptor is linked to the enzyme adenylcyclase which catalyses the conversation of ATP to cyclic AMP (Fig. 5.4), and so is responsible for initiating the appropriate biological effects.

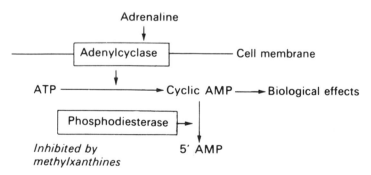

Fig. 5.4 The relationship of adenylcyclase to adrenaline activity.

Cyclic AMP is inactivated by conversion to 5' AMP under the influence of the enzyme phosphodiesterase. This enzyme can itself be inhibited by drugs of the methylxanthine group such as caffeine and theophylline, the effects of which, therefore, mimic sympathetic stimulation in many ways.

α-receptor agonists

Noradrenaline, a catecholamine, is the neurochemical mediator released by nerve impulses and various drugs from postganglionic sympathetic or 'adrenergic' neurones. It is predominantly an α-receptor stimulating drug, but also has β-stimulating properties which can best be demonstrated after α-receptor blockade. It produces an increase in systolic and diastolic blood pressures due to vasoconstriction of skin and splanchnic vessels. Compensatory vagal reflexes then slow the heart, masking a weak β-receptor mediated cardioaccelerator action. Peripheral resistance increases in most vascular beds resulting in a fall in blood flow through the kidney, brain, liver and splanchnic regions. Indications for its use are conditions of serious hypotension, but it must be emphasized that any increase in blood pressure produced by noradrenaline is at the expense of tissue perfusion. Toxic effects are the result of its pressor action and include headache, photophobia and vomiting, and the serious consequences of hypertension such as cerebral haemorrhage and pulmonary oedema.

Phenylephrine is a powerful α-receptor stimulating drug with only little β-receptor activity. Its effects on the cardiovascular system are similar to those of noradrenaline on α-receptors, with hypertension due to widespread vasoconstriction leading to reflex bradycardia. Renal and skin blood flows are reduced. Its absorption from the gastrointestinal tract is unreliable, and it is an unsatisfactory and inconsistent mydriatic, except in the presence of denervation where it produces a potentiated mydriasis. It is used in several nasal decongestant preparations because of its vasoconstrictor action.

β-receptor agonists

Isoprenaline is a catecholamine with potent β-receptor stimulating properties. It also has weak α-receptor stimulating properties, but these can only be shown on certain organs in the presence of β-blockade. It is a general β-stimulant and is not selective in its action on β_1 or β_2-receptors.

Cardiovascular effects. Isoprenaline increases cardiac output by positive inotropic and chronotropic actions, that is, it increases both the force and rate of myocardial contractions. It dilates coronary and skeletal muscle arteries, and to a lesser extent renal, mesenteric and skin blood vessels. This results in a fall in diastolic blood pressure, but because of the increased cardiac output, mean blood pressure may not fall to the same extent.

Respiratory system. Isoprenaline stimulates the respiratory centre, increasing the rate and depth of respiration. It is a potent bronchodilator, stimulating β-receptors in the bronchial musculature, and this is the basis for its widespread clinical use in bronchial asthma.

Other smooth muscle. Isoprenaline decreases the tone and motility of the musculature of the gastrointestinal tract, and inhibits uterine motility and tone.

Central nervous system. Isoprenaline produces central nervous stimulation with anxiety, restlessness and vomiting. Psychological dependence may develop in asthmatic patients treated for long periods with aerosol preparations. It also increases tremor and the rate of muscle contraction in reflexes.

Isoprenaline is absorbed sublingually and by aerosol but its absorption from the gastrointestinal tract is unpredictable. Unwanted effects include palpitations, tachycardia, dysrhythmias and anginal pain. Administration of large doses over long periods of time may produce myocardial necrosis in experimental animals.

Salbutamol is a sympathomimetic amine which acts preferentially on β_2-receptors to produce bronchodilatation and vasodilatation of skeletal muscle arterioles in doses which do not produce a significant increase in rate and force of cardiac contraction. In higher doses, however, cardiac effects are seen and tremor occurs. It is widely used in the treatment of bronchial asthma and is administered by inhalation, intravenous infusion or in tablet form.

Fenoterol, isoetharine, orciprenaline, reproterol, rimiterol and terbutaline are other selective β_2-agonists with similar properties to salbutamol.

Indications for β_2-agonists

Bronchial asthma (see Ch. 11).
Cardiac failure and heart block (see Ch. 8).
Premature labour (see Ch. 15).

Adrenaline

Adrenaline is produced by cells of the adrenal medulla and chromaffin tissue elsewhere in the body. It stimulates both α and β-adrenergic receptors throughout the body, its effects on different organs depending on the distribution of receptors within them.

Cardiovascular system. Adrenaline has a direct stimulating action on the heart mediated through its β-receptors, increasing the strength of ventricular contraction and the heart rate, and dilating coronary vessels. The response of blood vessels to adrenaline varies according to their α and β-receptor distribution. Arteriolar vessels in skin, mucosa and kidney are generally constricted by the action of α-receptors, but there are some vessels which dilate due to β-receptor stimulation in certain regions. Arterioles in skeletal muscles are dilated due to their β-receptors. The vasoconstrictor effects therefore tend to increase systemic blood pressure while the dilatation of skeletal vessels tends to decrease it.

Gastrointestinal tract. Its effects on the gut depend on initial tone and motility, but in general are to reduce tone and contract the pyloric and ileocaecal sphincters.

Respiratory system. Adrenaline has a brief stimulant effect on the respiratory centre, but this is not of therapeutic value. Its main effects are on β-receptors in the bronchial musculature producing relaxation which is most evident when the muscle is contracted due to disease such as bronchial asthma, to vagal stimulation or to drugs such as histamine or cholinergic agents. It also produces vasoconstriction in the bronchial mucosa to reduce vascularity and engorgement.

Eye. It has little effect on the pupil when applied locally, but in the sympathectomized eye, or following treatment with local guanethidine it produces marked mydriasis. Adrenaline lowers intraocular pressure in normal subjects and in glaucoma.

As adrenaline is rapidly destroyed in the gastrointestinal tract it must be given parenterally by the intramuscular or subcutaneous routes, or by inhalation.

Therapeutic uses

(a) Cardiac arrest.

(b) Anaphylactic shock, urticaria, angioneurotic oedema and serum sickness, when its subcutaneous administration gives prompt and dramatic relief. In anaphylactic shock adrenaline can be life saving, antagonizing histamine induced bronchoconstriction by β_2-receptor stimulation, and histamine induced vasodilatation and hypotension by α-receptor mediated vasoconstriction. In addition, it may inhibit further histamine release from mast cells by increasing intracellular cyclic AMP concentrations through β-receptor stimulation.

(c) In combination with local anaesthetics to limit their rate of absorption and provide a bloodless field of operation.

(d) Its use in bronchial asthma has been superseded by β_2-selective stimulant drugs.

Toxicity

The chief toxic effect of adrenaline is acute hypertension with its complications, particularly pulmonary oedema. Cardiac dysrhythmias may also occur, particularly during anaesthesia with halogenated hydrocarbon anaesthetics such as chloroform and halothane.

ADRENERGIC NEURONE BLOCKADE

Blockade of adrenergic neurone activity may be achieved in three ways.

(a) The release of noradrenaline by a nerve impulse is prevented, although noradrenaline depletion does not occur.

(b) Noradrenaline depletion occurs so that there is none available for release by a nerve impulse.

(c) Noradrenaline synthesis is impaired, or a false transmitter is substituted for noradrenaline with a weaker pressor action, so that sympathetic nerve activity results in a reduced pressor response.

Guanethidine

Guanethidine specifically blocks adrenergic neurone activity, by two distinct mechanisms.

(a) It prevents the release of noradrenaline in response to sympathetic nerve stimulation, even though noradrenaline stores remain intact. It is probable that this is the mechanism of its action responsible for its antihypertensive effect in therapeutic doses, for indirectly-acting amines such as tyramine still possess pressor and mydriatic activity in hypertensive patients treated with oral guanethidine.

(b) Higher concentrations of guanethidine, achieved for example by intravenous administration, produce depletion of noradrenaline from the adrenergic neurone by a release process which may result in an initial hypertensive effect before the blood pressure falls.

Similarly, the local instillation of guanethidine into the eye results in an initial mydriasis due to noradrenaline release before the appearance of miosis.

As with ganglion-blocking drugs, the antihypertensive effect depends on peripheral pooling with reduced venous return and cardiac output. Patients should be treated as far as possible in the upright posture rather than supine, and should be advised to avoid sudden changes in position and rate of movement to reduce the risk of postural hypotension. Guanethidine has a long half-life in the body and its action is slow to develop. It is administered in a single daily dose starting with 10 to 20 mg and increments should not be given more frequently than every 4 to 7 days. Tolerance may develop.

The commonest side-effects of treatment are diarrhoea and parotid pain. Nasal congestion, muscular weakness, fluid retention and failure of ejaculation may be troublesome. Rarely guanethidine produces mental depression.

Bethanidine

This antihypertensive drug has similar pharmacological properties to guanethidine, but is more rapidly excreted and its effects are therefore much shorter. It is administered in divided daily doses every 6 to 8 hours. Postural hypotension and the other side-effects of treatment with guanethidine may also be seen with bethanidine.

Debrisoquine

Like guanethidine and bethanidine in oral doses, debrisoquine produces adrenergic neurone blockade without noradrenaline depletion. Intravenous debrisoquine, however, produces a sharp rise in blood pressure, which is probably due to release of noradrenaline from adrenergic nerve endings. Side-effects are similar to those observed with guanethidine and bethanidine.

Interactions of guanethidine, bethanidine and debrisoquine are discussed on page 37.

Reserpine

Reserpine is an alkaloid obtained from the roots of *Rauwolfia serpentina*, a climbing shrub indigenous to India and neighbouring countries. It depletes tissues of noradrenaline, 5-hydroxytryptamine and dopamine. While its central tranquillizing activity is probably associated with changes in concentration of these amines in the brain, its antihypertensive effect is due largely to depletion of noradrenaline from adrenergic nerve endings in the heart and blood vessels. This leads to vasodilatation, reduced venous return and diminished cardiac output, while vagal predominance in the heart produces bradycardia.

The most serious side-effect of treatment with reserpine is mental depression which may be severe enough to cause suicidal attempts by some patients. This is seen particularly if the daily dose exceeds 0.3 mg, but successful antihypertensive therapy can usually be achieved by doses between 0.1 and 0.25 mg daily, given in a single oral dose because of its cumulative effect.

Depletion of brain dopamine by reserpine in large doses may produce Parkinsonism accompanied by choreoathetosis and cerebellar ataxia, and hyperprolactinaemia with galactorrhoea. Diarrhoea, nasal stuffiness, fluid retention with cardiac failure, and endocrine disturbances such as amenorrhoea, gynaecomastia, and impairment of sexual function have been described. Increased gastric secretion may lead to reactivation of peptic ulcer with the complications of haemorrhage and perforation. A report of an increased incidence of carcinoma of the breast in women treated with reserpine for hypertension has not been confirmed in several studies involving larger numbers of patients.

α-methyldopa

The mechanism of action of α-methyldopa is still obscure. It both inhibits the synthesis of noradrenaline and is itself converted into a false transmitter, α-methylnoradrenaline, which replaces noradrenaline in the sympathetic nerve ending. However, pharmacological studies with α-methylnoradrenaline in man and on human tissues have not provided conclusive evidence that it is a weaker pressor agent than noradrenaline. Indeed, there is evidence in animals that α-methylnoradrenaline is a more potent agonist than noradrenaline at central presynaptic adrenergic α-receptors which regulate sympathetic outflow (p. 70); stimulation of these receptors leads to a reduction in peripheral sympathetic tone. Premedication with a selective α-receptor blocking drug such as phentolamine prevents this action.

Whereas the effects of guanethidine, bethanidine and debrisoquine are seen predominantly in the erect position, and postural hypotension as a common side-effect of treatment, α-methyldopa reduces blood pressure in both recumbent and upright positions.

The most common side-effect of treatment with α-methyldopa is sedation, probably due to depletion of noradrenaline from the brain. It tends to disappear with continued administration of the drug, but withdrawal of treatment after a long period of administration may result in the appearance of a state of excitement with restlessness and insomnia. Like the other adrenergic neurone-blocking drugs it may cause bradycardia, stuffy nose, failure of ejaculation, and sodium and water retention with oedema and cardiac failure. A positive antiglobulin (Coomb's) test has been found in 20% of patients taking α-methyldopa, but clinical evidence of haemolysis is rare.

ADRENERGIC RECEPTOR BLOCKADE

Drugs which prevent or interfere with the release of noradrenaline from the adrenergic neurone block sympathetic activity irrespective of whether the nerve is supplying α or β-receptors and the result is a general reduction in sympathetic activity. Those now to be discussed act at the receptor site, blocking the effects of noradrenaline and other directly-acting amines oneither α or β-receptors. In general, they are most effective against circulating catecholamines than against those endogenously derived from neurotransmitter stores in the body.

α-adrenergic receptor blocking drugs

Phenoxybenzamine and dibenamine

These drugs are chemically related to the nitrogen mustards and are alkylating agents. They are highly reactive and have other pharmacological actions than simple α-adrenergic receptor blockade, including blockade of histamine and 5-hydroxytryptamine on smooth muscle. Small doses produce sedation probably due to their α-adrenergic blocking action, but high doses produce central nervous stimulation with nausea, vomiting, hyperventilation and convulsions.

The effects of α-adrenergic receptor blockade in therapeutic doses are chiefly seen in the cardiovascular system, where a small fall in diastolic pressure occurs with a compensatory tachycardia. If the plasma volume is reduced, however, or if hypertension is present, a marked fall in blood pressure may occur, which is greater in the erect than a supine position. These drugs may be administered orally or parenterally and adrenergic blockade may persist for up to 3 to 4 days.

Tolazoline

This is a competitive inhibitor of α-adrenergic receptor activity, and also of 5-hydroxytryptamine. In addition it has a direct relaxant action on smooth muscle and intrinsic sympathomimetic (partial agonist) activity including cardiac stimulation. It has cholinergic effects on the gastrointestinal tract which are blocked by atropine, and histamine-like actions such as stimulation of gastric secretion. Its effects on the cardiovascular system are, therefore, complex and depend on several types of action. Side effects include flushing, tachycardia, dysrhythmias, anginal pain, nausea, vomiting, diarrhoea and exacerbation of peptic ulcer.

Phentolamine

Phentolamine resembles tolazoline in possessing other marked pharmacological effects besides its α-receptor blocking properties. In particular it has potent smooth muscle relaxing effects, and intrinsic sympathomimetic activity. The first may lead to a profound reduction in blood pressure and so produce a false positive in the 'Rogitine test' for diagnosis of a phaeochromocytoma. This test depends on producing a fall in blood pressure with intravenous phentolamine in patients in whom hypertension is due to a phaeochromocytoma. It has, however, been superseded by direct measurement of urinary or plasma catecholamines or their metabolites. The intrinsic sympathomimetic activity includes cardiac stimulation, and palpitations and tachycardia may be distressing following intravenous administration. Other side-effects include nasal congestion, nausea, vomiting and diarrhoea.

Thymoxamine

Thymoxamine is a competitive α-receptor blocking drug with relatively few other important pharmacological actions, which include weak antihistamine effects. It produces miosis when applied locally to the eye, and a rise in skin temperature when applied in a water-free cetomacrogol base, due to reduction in α-receptor-mediated vasoconstriction in the skin leading to an increase in cutaneous blood flow. A fall in systemic blood pressure, particularly marked in the erect position, occurs after intravenous administration, and also after large oral doses. It has a very short plasma half-life, however, and its absorption after oral administration is erratic.

Indoramin

This has recently been introduced as an antihypertensive drug. Its action in therapeutic doses appears to depend largely on α-receptor blockade although in higher concentrations myocardial depression may occur. It also has antihistamine properties. Sedation commonly occurs.

Prazosin

When first introduced as an antihypertensive agent, prazosin was thought to act primarily through direct smooth muscle relaxation. It is now believed to be a competitive α-adrenoceptor blocking drug which also possesses some direct relaxant properties. It lowers blood pressure by producing dilatation particularly of resistance arterioles. Dizziness and headaches may occur with its use, but its most important adverse effect is a transient loss of consciousness associated with profound hypotension which, while it most commonly occurs at the start of treatment, may also occur at other times, and the exact cause of which is not yet understood. Patients treated with prazosin should be kept under observation for some hours after receiving the first dose, which should always be small.

Ergot

Ergot alkaloids were the first adrenergic blocking drugs to be discovered by the classical studies of Dale in 1906. Most of their pharmacological and therapeutic actions are due to properties other than adrenergic blockade, however, and the true nature of their activity is not yet known in detail. They have a direct stimulant action on smooth muscle, which may in fact be a sympathomimetic action. This is responsible for the rise in blood pressure which ergot preparations produce, and for the coronary vasoconstriction which may occur and cause marked ischaemia in patients with coronary artery disease. Prolonged administration may cause vascular insufficiency and gangrene of the extremities.

Indications for α-receptor blockade

Although α-adrenergic receptor blocking drugs are widely prescribed for a variety of conditions, their proven value is limited to a few well-defined situations.

Phaeochromocytoma. While of doubtful value in the diagnosis of this condition, α-receptor blockade is indicated in the preoperative and operative management of the established case, where it prevents the paroxysmal hypertension which characterizes the condition and which is particularly likely to occur during operative manipulation of the tumour. Phenoxybenzamine is most often used, and is given orally preoperatively and intravenously for 12 hours before and during surgery.

Essential hypertension. Phenoxybenzamine and phentolamine have little place in the management of essential hypertension, largely due to their other unwanted and unpleasant pharmacological actions. Prazosin and indoramin, however, are now established in the management of hypertensive patients who have not been controlled with combined diuretic + β-adrenoceptor blocking drug or diuretic + methyldopa treatment, and in whom the addition of an α-receptor blocking drug may produce a further fall in blood pressure. Tachycardia seldom occurs with antihypertensive doses, but should a reflex increase in heart rate accompany their vaso-dilating effects, this will be reduced or prevented by the accompanying administration of a β-receptor blocking drug.

Shock. In the past it has been part of the standard treatment of cardiovascular shock to administer sympathomimetic pressor agents such as noradrenaline to increase blood pressure, even though the effect of these drugs has been to reduce blood flow to organs such as the kidneys and gut. This is particularly dangerous in conditions such as haemorrhage, trauma or infection where hypovolaemia may be present. There is evidence that the best way to treat such conditions is to induce vasodilatation by inhibiting sympathetic vasoconstriction with α-receptor blocking drugs or by directly relaxing vascular smooth muscle, together with expansion of the plasma volume with blood or other suitable fluids.

Peripheral vascular disease. Although the α-receptor blocking drugs phenoxybenzamine, tolazoline and thymoxamine have been widely used in peripheral vascular disease, their real value has yet to be established. There is evidence that in intermittent claudication blood may actually be shunted away from the ischaemic limb to normal areas because of vasodilatation in them. Vasodilatation in skeletal muscle arterioles is β-receptor mediated, and it is therefore unlikely that α-receptor blocking drugs would be effective in claudication. On theoretical grounds ischaemic conditions of the skin are the most likely form of peripheral vascular disease to be helped by these drugs, but confirmation in clinical trials is not yet available.

β-adrenergic receptor blocking drugs

In general, β-adrenergic receptor blocking drugs are structurally similar to the β-adrenergic agonist drugs such as isoprenaline. The first of this class to be introduced was dichloroisoprenaline (DCI) which blocked those responses to adrenaline and other sympathomimetic amines which involve β-receptors, but also had intrinsic agonist activity of its own comparable to that of isoprenaline. As a result it was not of clinical value. Pronethalol was more suitable for clinical use as it had considerably less intrinsic activity than DCI, but repeated administration to mice over a long period of time appeared to have carcinogenic effects and it was, therefore, withdrawn.

There are now several potent β-receptor blocking drugs which differ in certain properties such as partial agonist (or intrinsic sympathomimetic) activity, membrane stabilizing activity, and selectivity of action at different β-receptors (Table 5.2). In general, however, they have the following effects:

Table 5.2 Comparative properties of β-adrenoceptor blocking drugs

Drug	Selectivity for B_1 receptors	Partial agonist activity	Membrane stabilizing activity
Acebutolol	+	+	+
Alprenolol	−	+	+
Atenolol	+	−	−
Betaxolol	+	−	±
Metoprolol	+	−	−
Nadolol	−	−	−
Oxprenolol	−	+	+
Pindolol	−	+	+
Practolol	+	+	−
Propranolol	−	−	+
Sotalol	−	−	−
Timolol	−	?	−

Cardiovascular system. β-receptor blocking drugs, such as propranolol, produce a fall in heart rate, cardiac output, arterial pressure and left ventricular minute work. During exercise the effects are much greater, with reduction of the normal increment of heart rate, cardiac output, mean arterial pressure and left ventricular minute work, and an increase in the arterio-mixed venous oxygen difference. Propranolol is a racemic mixture of (+)- and (−)-isomers, and it appears that the β-receptor blocking properties reside predominantly in the (−) isomer. In higher concentrations propranolol has direct membrane-stabilizing or 'quinidine-like' effects on the myocardium.

Respiratory system. Sympathetically induced bronchodilatation is mediated by the β-adrenergic receptors, and their blockade by β-blocking drugs may, therefore, lead to an increase in airways resistance. This may be particularly harmful to patients with bronchial asthma, chronic bronchitis, or other forms of respiratory insufficiency. A number of β-blocking drugs have been developed which appear to possess certain degrees of selectivity of action, blocking β_1-receptors in the heart at lower concentrations than the β_2-receptors in the bronchi. Practolol is the most cardioselective of these drugs, but had to be withdrawn from general clinical use because it produced a syndrome comprising psoriasiform rashes, dry eyes, progressing to more serious ophthalmic changes, and sclerosing peritonitis, sometimes associated with antinuclear factor. Acebutolol, atenolol, betaxolol and metoprolol are other 'cardioselective' drugs which are in therapeutic use. Their cardioselectivity is, however, only relative, and in the oral therapeutic doses normally used in hypertension and angina, they may produce clinically important increases in airways resistance. Their advantage over non-selective drugs such as alprenolol, nadolol, propranolol, oxprenolol, pindolol, sotalol and timolol appears to be that their bronchoconstricting action can be more readily overcome by administration of a β_2 agonist drug such as rimiterol, salbutamol or terbutaline. Some β-blocking drugs, including alprenolol, oxprenolol and pindolol are partial agonists, having a receptor stimulant as well as blocking action, and there is evidence that this property may confer some advantage over drugs without it in patients with asthma. However, it must be emphasized that all β-blocking drugs may precipitate asthmatic attacks in patients with this condition, and they are, therefore, contraindicated in such patients.

Nervous system. There is evidence that the central control of blood pressure is influenced by central α- and β-adrenoceptor activity, stimulation of central α-receptors producing a fall in blood pressure, and stimulation of central β-receptors a rise in blood pressure. Central β-blockade might, therefore, produce a fall in sympathetic outflow and systemic blood pressure (p. 70), but there is little evidence that this contributes to the antihypertensive effect of β-blocking drugs. Central nervous adverse effects occur quite frequently with these drugs, however, including sleep disturbances, dreams, hypnogogic hallucinations, lethargy, sedation and depression. Propranolol has also been claimed to possess anti-psychotic effects in high doses such as 1–2 g daily, about ten times the usual dose for other indications. Such central actions are not necessarily due to β-receptor blockade, for these drugs also possess potent central 5HT antagonist properties which might account for some of these effects. Furthermore, brain cell concentrations of propranolol achieved with the high doses of propranolol used in antipsychotic treatment might be associated with direct membrane-stabilizing activity. If such an antipsychotic action exists, however, it is more probable that the mechanism is pharmacokinetic as administration of propranolol has been shown to increase blood levels of neuroleptic drugs already being taken by the psychotic patients studied.

Isoprenaline and adrenaline increase tremor by a direct action on skeletal muscle, and this may be prevented by β-receptor blocking drugs, although it is uncertain whether this is entirely due to peripheral blockade or whether there is a cental component to their anti-tremor action. It appears that tremor is mediated mainly through β_2-receptors.

Eye. Some β-blocking drugs, such as propranolol, which posses local anaesthetic properties produce marked corneal anaesthesia when instilled into the eye, and have been used surgically for this purpose.

Intraocular pressure may, paradoxically, be reduced by both α- and β-adrenoceptor agonists and antagonists because of their different actions on aqueous production and reabsorption. Most β-blocking drugs reduce intraocular pressure, at least transiently, and timolol appears to have a sustained ocular hypotensive action which is being widely exploited in the treatment of glaucoma. Even when timolol is instilled into the conjunctival sac for this purpose, however, sufficient may be absorbed systemically to produce the cardiovascular and other effects of β-receptor blockade.

Drugs with both α- and β-receptor blocking properties

It is possible that some β-blocking drugs possess minor α-adrenoceptor blocking properties. Labetalol, however, combines α- and β-receptor blocking activity in a ratio of about 1:5 and is an effective antihypertensive agent, particularly when used intravenously to control severe hypertension. Adverse effects include postural hypotension, bronchoconstriction, nasal stuffiness, vivid dreams, epigastric pain and itching of the scalp.

Indications for β-receptor blockade

Angina. Coronary vasodilatation is mediated by β-receptor activity, and β-blockade may produce a fall in coronary flow. However, the reduction in cardiac work and oxygen requirements which it produces, particularly during exercise or emotional states, may be greater than its effects on coronary flow, and so the use of propranolol and other β-blocking drugs has proved to be of value in many cases of angina pectoris. Large doses are required in many patients, however, in excess of those needed to block exogenously administered isoprenaline, and it is possible, therefore, that other mechanisms of action may be involved.

Cardiac dysrhythmias. β-Receptor blocking drugs prevent or abolish catecholamine-induced dysrhythmias in experimental animals and man, and are of value in the management of patients with phaeochromocytoma at risk from ventricular dysrhythmias. They may also abolish digitalis-induced dysrhythmias, the mechanism of this being uncertain.

Hypertension. β-Receptor blocking drugs have significant antihypertensive effects which may be seen when used alone or in combination with other antihypertensive drugs or thiazide diuretics. This action is not yet fully understood, but may involve several factors including (a) blockade of central β-receptors involved in blood pressure control and sympathetic outflow (p. 70); (b) inhibition of renin production in the kidney, which is mediated, at least in part, by β-adrenergic activity, with an associated fall in angiotensin generation and aldosterone secretion; (c) a fall in cardiac output, although this may be followed by a reflex increase in peripheral resistance; (d) an influence on baroreceptor activity; (e) blockade of presynaptic β-receptors may lead to a decrease of noradrenaline release in response to sympathetic nervous activity and therefore to a reduction in postsynaptic adrenoceptor stimulation (p. 53); (f) increased vasodilator prostaglandin activity. Consistent with this is the antagonistic effect of indomethacin on the antihypertensive effects of β-blocking drugs (page 42).

Phaeochromocytoma. When α-receptors are blocked with phenoxybenzamine, catecholamines produced by the tumour can still produce an increase in heart rate or a dysrhythmia by β-receptor stimulation. This occurs irrespective of whether adrenaline or noradrenaline is the predominant catecholamine secreted by the tumour. These effects can be prevented or abolished by a β-receptor blocking drug such as propranolol, given by mouth in the preoperative period after commencement of treatment with an α-receptor blocking drug, and intravenously during operative removal of the tumour.

Hyperthyroidism. Many of the peripheral manifestations of hyperthyroidism are due to increased β-receptor activity and may be reduced by β-blocking drugs. In this condition there is also increased responsiveness to adrenergic stimulation, however, and therefore those drugs which possess intrinsic agonist activity are not so effective as those without it such as propranolol and sotalol.

Anxiety. Autonomic activity, particularly sympathetic, is prominent in anxiety states, and propranolol has been shown to significantly reduce the physical symptomatology of patients with this condition. Its effects are particularly seen where complaints of palpitations and tachycardia are prominent, but may also relieve other autonomic effects such as sweating and diarrhoea.

Tremor. β-blocking drugs reduce both physiological and essential tremor by a direct action on skeletal muscle. This is probably a β_2-mediated effect.

Migraine. Propranolol has been shown to be of prophylactic value in reducing the incidence and severity of migraine attacks in some patients. This property is not shared by all β-blockers, and in particular by those with partial agonist properties, such as oxprenolol and pindolol. The mechanism is not yet understood.

Glaucoma (see p. 66)

Portal hypertension. There is some evidence that administration of propranolol to patients with oesophageal varices secondary to hepatic cirrhosis may reduce the risk or severity of bleeding from the varices. The mechanism is not clear but may involve a fall in portal venous pressure.

Untoward effects of β-receptor blockade.

Cardiovascular. β-blocking drugs may precipitate or make worse cardiac failure, due to withdrawal of cardiac sympathetic drive, and they should be used with great caution in patients with reduced cardiac reserve. They may also exacerbate Raynaud's phenomenon and produce cold extremities, due to unopposed cutaneous α-receptor vasoconstriction.

Respiratory. These have already been discussed (p. 65).

Central nervous. Sleep disturbance, nightmares, hallucinations, and depression occur rarely (p. 66).

Others. Potentiation of the hypoglycaemic action of insulin and sulphonylurea antidiabetic drugs may occur. The practolol syndrome which lead to its withdrawal has already been discussed (p. 65).

IIYPERTENSION

The role of adrenergic receptor blocking drugs in the treatment of phaeochromocytoma has already been discussed. In forms of hypertension due to other known pathological causes, and in essential hypertension, drugs which influence sympathetic control of the heart and blood vessels, and drugs which influence vascular tone by other mechanisms may be effective in reducing blood pressure, even though increased sympathetic tone may not be primarily responsible for the condition. Sites at which drugs may interfere with sympathetic activity in the management of hypertension are shown in Figure 5.5.

1. The afferent neurone

The veratrum alkaloids interfere with afferent autonomic neurone activity, particularly from pressure and stretch receptors in the heart and carotid-sinus baroreceptor areas, resulting in a reduction in sympathetic outflow from the hypothalamus. They have marked toxic effects, however, and are not used clinically.

2. Cortical function

Anxiety and emotional stress may be associated with increases in blood pressure, and although these may only be transient there is evidence that they may lead to persistent hypertension in the future. Although of little value in the management of essential hypertension, sedative and tranquillizing drugs such as benzodiazepines may reduce tension and anxiety and prevent excessive increases in blood pressure in response to stress.

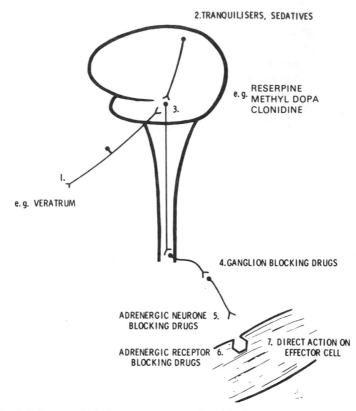

Fig. 5.5 Sites at which drugs may act to reduce blood pressure.

3. Hypothalamus

Several antihypertensive drugs, including reserpine, α-methyldopa
and clonidine, produce sedation as unwanted effects, and it is probable that this is due to actions on central neurotransmitters.
Sympathetic tone on the heart and blood vessels is regulated by
cardio-acceleratory and vasomotor centres in the hypothalamus and
brain stem. There is animal evidence that the activity of these
centres is influenced by central noradrenergic and adrenergic α- and
β-receptor activity. Central α-receptor stimulation is associated with
a fall in sympathetic outflow, which can be blocked by pretreatment
with a specific α-blocking drug such as phentolamine. Central β-
receptor activity, on the other hand, appears to produce an increase
in sympathetic outflow. It is probable that α-methyldopa (p. 59)
and clonidine (p. 72) owe their antihypertensive effects, at least in

part, to central α-receptor stimulation. While it is tempting to postulate that some of the antihypertensive action of propranolol and other β-blocking drugs depends on central β-receptor blockade, there is no good evidence for this.

4. Autonomic ganglia

Drugs blocking autonomic ganglia have already been discussed. Because of their erratic absorption from the gut, and the unpleasant effects of general autonomic blockade which they produce, their use is restricted to the treatment of hypertensive emergencies, where they are administered parenterally until the blood pressure is brought under control.

5. Adrenergic neurone

The actions of guanethidine, bethanidine, debrisoquine and reserpine have already been discussed (pp. 57–58). Their use is decreasing, largely because of their adverse effects and the important interactions of the first three with monoamine reuptake inhibiting drugs (p. 37).

6. Adrenergic receptor

α-adrenergic receptor blocking drugs are useful in the management of phaeochromocytoma. Although earlier non-competitive drugs, such as phenoxybenzamine, have little place in essential hypertension, the competitive α-blocking drugs prazosin and indoramin, appear to be of value in some patients with essential hypertension who have failed to respond adequately to first-line treatment (p. 63). β-receptor blocking drugs are now considered by many physicians to be the firstline treatment in essential hypertension as well as in protecting the myocardium from the effects of excess catecholamines in patients with phaeochromocytomata. Labetalol, which combines α- and β-adrenoceptor blocking activity is particularly valuable when administered intravenously in management of severely hypertensive patients.

7. Drugs acting directly on the vascular smooth muscle

Thiazide diuretics and other related compounds such as indapamide and xipamide have an antihypertensive action which may be effective in sub-diuretic doses and does not appear to depend simply on reduction in extracellular fluid volume and cardiac output. They may have a direct action on the blood vessel wall, reducing its sensitivity to catecholamines, angiotensin and other pressor substances by mechanisms beyond the adrenoceptor. They may be used alone in the management of essential hypertension, or may be used together with other drugs such as β-antagonists, α-methyldopa and more potent vasodilators. The doses of the latter may, therefore, be reduced with a consequent reduction in incidence of adverse effects and cost of treatment. Plasma potassium concentrations should be monitored in patients requiring digitalis treatment for atrial fibrillation or cardiac failure (p. 143).

Diazoxide is a thiazide drug without diuretic activity, but with marked hyperglycaemic and hypotensive effects. It is given by intravenous administration in acute hypertensive emergencies while treatment with an oral agent is substituted.

Hydralazine probably owes its antihypertensive action predominantly to a generalised direct relaxation of vascular smooth muscle. It became unpopular because of its undesirable effects, the most common being headache, palpitations, tachycardia, angina, anorexia, nausea and vomiting. More dangerous are bone marrow depression, an acute rheumatoid state, and rarely, a syndrome resembling systemic lupus erythematosus. However, it has regained some popularity as a second-line treatment of essential hypertension in patients already receiving a β-adrenoceptor blocking drug together with a thiazide-type drug but with inadequate blood pressure control. The addition of relatively small doses of hydralazine may achieve satisfactory levels of blood pressure with little risk of adverse effects, tachycardia and angina seldom occurring in the presence of β-blockade. Endralazine, a related drug, is now being assessed clinically. It appears to have a lower incidence of S.L.E. type reactions, and does not depend on acetylator status for its rate of metabolism as does hydralazine (page 19).

Minoxidil is a highly-potent vasodilator which may be efective in patients whose blood pressure has not been controlled with other drugs. Its major adverse effect is increased hair growth which can be distressing particularly in women. Fluid retention and tachycardia frequently occur, and a diuretic such as frusemide and a β-blocker are usually given together with minoxidil.

Clonidine is a potent antihypertensive drug whose mode of action is not yet clearly understood. While there is some evidence for a central action (p. 70), it has peripheral effects on blood vessels, reducing their response both to the constrictor effect of noradrenaline and to the dilator action of isoprenaline. Sedation, depression and dryness of the mouth occur, but its most important adverse effect is rebound hypertension associated with sudden termination of long-term therapy, the pharmacological mechanism of which is not yet known.

Calcium antagonists such as nifedipine. Contraction of vascular smooth muscle depends upon an influx of calcium ions into the muscle cell through the cell membrane. More than one calcium channel through the membrane is thought to exist, and one of these is blocked by nifedipine and other so-called calcium antagonists such as verapamil (page 152). Nifedipine is a potent peripheral vasodilator and is being assessed not only in treatment of hypertension but also of migraine and peripheral vascular disease. Its principal unwanted effects are flushing and headaches.

Angiotension-converting enzyme (ACE) inhibitors such as captopril, mediate the conversion of angiotensin I to angiotensin II. It is a logical step, therefore, to develop drugs such as captopril that inhibit this enzyme and reduce angiotensin II production, particularly in patients with renal hypertension in whom this pathway plays an important pathogenic role. While captopril is certainly of value to such patients, it also has profound hypotensive effects in patients without renal disease, and in whom there is no evidence of high renin or angiotensin I status. The mechanisms of all its antihypertensive effects are not yet understood. Its usefulness is limited by its unwanted effects which include loss of taste, proteinuria, bone marrow depression and hyperkalaemia.

In its early clinical trials its use was markedly limited by these unwanted effects. More recently, however, it has been found to have antihypertensive effects at much lower doses than in the early trials, and the incidence of unwanted effects has been greatly reduced. It may produce fluid retention, and a loop diuretic is usually co-prescribed with it. The chemical structure of captopril contains a sulphydryl group (-S-H-), as does that of penicillamine, and it may be that this explains some of the unwanted effects of these drugs, particularly the loss of taste, proteinuria and bone-marrow effects. Another ACE inhibitor, enalopril, has recently been introduced which does not contain the sulphydryl group in its chemical structure, and its therapeutic and adverse effect profiles are being assessed.

Pargyline is a monoamine oxidase inhibitor. These drugs have paradoxical effects on blood pressure. Their hypertensive complications associated with the ingestion of tyramine-containing food-stuffs have already been discussed. Postural hypotension has been noted with several of these drugs, although the mechanism is unknown, and pargyline is the most consistent in its antihypertensive effects. However, it shares with the other drugs of this group the dangers of hypertensive crises, and also tends to promote fluid retention. It may unmask psychotic symptoms such as hallucinations and delusions.

Sodium nitroprusside, given by carefully monitored intravenous infusion, has a direct dilator effect on vascular musculature independent of neural mechanisms. The effect is immediate, and ends as soon as the infusion is stopped. It is, therefore, of particular value in the management of very severe hypertension or its acute complications. It has few if any short-term toxic effects. Long-term effects are due to accumulation of thiocyanate to which nitroprusside is converted, and serum levels should , therefore, be measured at frequent intervals.

Stepwise treatment of essential hypertension

High blood pressure requires treatment because it is an important risk factor in cardiovascular, cerebrovascular and renal diseases. Drugs should only be used when other factors such as obesity, high salt and alcohol intake and smoking habits have been corrected. If drug treatment is indicated, a stepwise approach is often used, only proceeding to a further step if response to the first step drugs is unsatisfactory when assessed in adequate dosage for an adequate period which is not usually less than two weeks.

Step 1. This is either a thiazide diuretic or a β-adrenoceptor blocking drug used alone. Personal preference of the physician usually decides which will be prescribed, but a history of gout or diabetes might contraindicate a thiazide, while a history of obstructive airways disease, cardiac failure or peripheral vascular disease might contraindicate a β-blocker.

Step 2 consists of combined treatment with a diuretic plus a β-blocker. Where either a diuretic a β-blocker are contraindicated, methyldopa might be considered, or an α-adrenoceptor blocking drug such as indoramin or prazosin.

Step 3 consists of addition of a vasodilator drug to the combination of diuretic plus β-blocker. A wide choice is now available including the α-blocking drugs (indoramin and prazosin), hydralazine, and the calcium antagonists (nifedipine).

Step 4 is reserved for patients in whom aggressive therapy through the first three steps has not produced acceptable control of blood pressure. Such patients require detailed investigation to exclude an underlying renal or endocrine cause for their hypertension. Depending on its severity and evidence of end-organ damage, potent vasodilators such as minoxidil or sodium nitroprusside may be used.

The place of ACE inhibitors such as captopril or enalapril in the management of essential hypertension is still being assessed. They may find a place as first or second-line choice of drugs for this indication as well as for the more specific uncommon indication of renal hypertension.

5-HYDROXYTRYPTAMINE

5-Hydroxytryptamine (5HT, serotonin) is widely distributed throughout the body, being concentrated in blood platelets and enterochromaffin cells of the gastrointestinal mucosa, which constitute the main storage sites of the body. It is synthesized from dietary tryptophan which is hydroxylated to 5-hydroxytryptophan (5HTP) and then decarboxylated to 5HT. Tumours of enterochromaffin cells, known as carcinoid tumours, produce excess of 5HT which contributes in part to the clinical picture of the condition.

5HT has a powerful vasoconstrictor effect which is direct and does not appear to involve nervous mechanisms. It also has strong contracting effects on various parts of the gastrointestinal tract. There is good evidence that 5HT is a transmitter in the central nervous systems (p. 78). Tissue levels are depleted by *p*-chlorophenylalanine which inhibits its synthesis, and reserpine which prevents its intracellular binding and thus leads to its destruction by monoamine oxidase.

5HT antagonists

Methysergide is a potent 5HT receptor blocking drug with partial agonist activity, which is used in the symptomatic treatment of the carcinoid syndrome and in the prophylaxis of migraine (p. 98). A large number of adverse effects are associated with its use, including vomiting, abdominal cramps and diarrhoea. Severe peripheral vasoconstriction may also occur. More serious is the production of retroperitoneal fibrosis in patients treated for longer periods of time, and it is advisable to restrict its administration to periods of not more than 3 months.

Cyproheptadine antagonizes the action of 5HT and also of other pharmacological substances such as histamine and acetylcholine. It has other interesting actions such as stimulation of appetite leading to an increase in body weight, and is sometimes used clinically for this purpose. Drowsiness occurs commonly with its use, and its anticholinergic effects may lead to dryness of the mouth, and precipitation of glaucoma or urinary retention in predisposed patients.

Ketanserin is a potent 5HT antagonist which is an effective antihypertensive drug. This was claimed as evidence for a possible role of 5HT in essential hypertension, but ketanserin has subsequently been shown also to possess marked α-adrenoceptor blocking properties which are probably responsible for its antihypertensive effects.

6

Neuropharmacology

CNS TRANSMITTERS AND DRUG ACTION

Less is known about the transmitters in the brain and spinal cord than in the peripheral nervous system simply because of the complexity and inaccessibility of these structures. For this reason it is usually more difficult to explain the effects of a centrally-acting drug in terms of modification of transmitter action, although there are a growing number of examples where this is now possible. With other drugs little more than an inspired guess can be made about their mode of action. If a chemical substance is to be considered as a putative transmitter in the central nervous system (CNS), it must satisfy several criteria: (a) it must occur naturally in the tissue, and be released by electrical stimulation, (b) enzymes for its synthesis and breakdown must be present, (c) local application or injection of the substance should mimic the action of the transmitter and (d) drugs which block synaptic transmission at this site should also block the effect of the locally-applied substance. Based on animal experiments, a number of substances satisfy these criteria either fully or in part.

Acetylcholine

This is found in considerable amounts in the tegmental pathways, cerebral cortex and basal ganglia, and is released from the cortex by electrical stimulation. Some cortical cells are excited by acetylcholine, while others are inhibited. Atropine can produce lack of concentration and memory, hallucinations and EEG alerting, and anticholinergic drugs used in Parkinsonism not infrequently precipitate toxic confusional states. A deficiency of acetylcholine and its synthetic enzyme, choline acetylase, has been demonstrated in Alzheimer's disease although attempts at correcting the deficiency by administering anticholinesterases or supplementing the intake of choline have so far been unsuccessful in producing symptomatic improvement.

Noradrenaline

This is most abundant in nerve fibres in the hypothalamus, median eminence, olfactory bulb, limbic system, cranial nerve nuclei, and the spinal cord. These nerve fibres arise almost exclusively from cell bodies in the lower brain stem, particularly in the pons, medulla and reticular formation. Drugs which modify noradrenergic transmission, such as monoamine oxidase inhibitors (MAOI), imipramine, amphetamine and reserpine, have marked effects on mood, motor activity, endocrine secretion from the pituitary, and body temperature. Circulating noradrenaline cannot cross the 'blood-brain barrier' (an anatomically ill-defined barrier which has the properties of a lipid membrane between the plasma and brain) but when injected into the cerebral ventricles it produces sedation.

Dopamine

In some nerve terminals the synthetic pathway producing catecholamines stops short at dopamine, and this substances appears to be the transmitter. Its importance in the neostriatum is established; degeneration of the nigro-striatal pathway, whose nerve terminals contain dopamine, leads to Parkinsonism. In addition, drugs which can block dopamine receptors, e.g. phenothiazines and butyrophenones, can produce Parkinsonism. Dopamine is involved in the inhibitory control of prolactin secretion from the anterior pituitary; drugs that block dopamine receptors cause hyper-prolactinaemia.

5-Hydroxytryptamine

This substance is found in highest concentrations in the anterior part of the hypothalamus and amygdala. Fibres which contain 5HT arise mainly from cells in the midline raphe nuclei of the brain stem. Electrical stimulation of these nuclei produces alerting in experimental animals. On the other hand, a lesion destroying these fibres can produce insomnia. 5HT is synthesized from tryptophan as follows:

Tryptophan → 5-hydroxytryptophan → 5-hydroxytryptamine

    hydroxylation   decarboxylation

Histamine

This can be found in synaptic vesicles in the hypothalamus, thalamus and cerebral cortex, although its possible role as a transmitter is undetermined.

Inhibitory amino acids

There are several of these substances, the most importance being γ-aminobutyric acid (GABA) and glycine. The former is restricted in its distribution to the central nervous system, and is present in larger amounts than any of the other amino acids. It acts as a postsynaptic inhibitory transmitter in the cerebral and cerebellar cortex, whereas in the spinal cord it mediates presynaptic inhibition of afferent pathways. Inhibitors of GABA-transaminase, the enzyme that degrades GABA, have anticonvulsant activity. Glycine is found particularly in the nerve terminals of spinal interneurones, and probably acts as a postsynaptic inhibitory transmitter on motoneurones.

Excitatory amino acids

The most widespread in their distribution are L-glutamic and L-aspartic acids. They are released from the cerebral cortex when the reticular formation is stimulated electrically. They excite many different types of nerve cell, including cortical neurones and spinal motoneurones.

Opioid peptides

These are found mainly in the sensory system (e.g. the substantia gelatinosa in the spinal cord), and in the autonomic, limbic and neuroendocrine systems where they operate as part of a widespread inhibitory system. They comprise a large group of related compounds which are subdivided into three families, encephalins, dynorphins and endorphins, and are derived from larger peptide molecules by enzyme cleavage; they are related to corticotrophin and β-lipotrophin. They function in some sites as short acting neurotransmitters and at others as long acting modulator neurohormones. The enkephalins are the most widely distributed and play an important part in neurotransmission in the pain pathways (p. 132). Opioid peptides are involved in autonomic reflexes under conditions of stress, e.g. anaesthesia, surgery, shock, pain, and they modulate the release of various hypothalamic-pituitary hormones.

Prostaglandins

Types E and F are widely distributed in the CNS and can produce a variety of effects when injected intravenously or applied directly to nerve cells, but a transmitter function has yet to be established for these substances.

Other putative neurotransmitters

Many other substances have been identified in the CNS which appear to satisfy some or all of the criteria demanded of a transmitter. These include substance P, vasoactive intestinal polypeptide, somatostatin, angiotensin and cholecystokinin, all of which are contained in afferent terminals in the spinal cord. In addition, the substantia gelatinosa contains neurotensin, neurophysin, oxytocin, glucagon, vasopressin, motilin and bombesin. A transmitter or modulator role is likely for at least some of these.

Modification of transmission

The central synapses which have been studied in greatest detail are those at which monoamines (noradrenaline, dopamine and 5HT) are the transmitters. The synthesis, release and fate of noradrenaline at the sympathetic postganglionic nerve terminal have been described in the last chapter. Central noradrenergic terminals are functionally similar to these. Figure 6.1 illustrates the sites at which some commonly used centrally-acting drugs modify transmission in these terminals. They can act in the following ways:

By modifying synthesis of monoamines (Site 1). The actions of α-methyl p-tyrosine and α-methyldopa on sympathetic nerve terminals are described on pages 48 and 59. Both can affect catecholamine synthesis in the brain leading to sedation, and α-methyl dopa occasionally produces depression in patients treated with this drug for hypertension.

Levodopa is given to patients with Parkinson's disease with the object of building up the depleted levels of dopamine in the corpus striatum. Levodopa (L-dopa) is identical to the naturally occurring dopa which is produced in the synthetic pathway for catecholamines (see p. 47). L-tryptophan, precursor to 5HT, increases 5HT levels

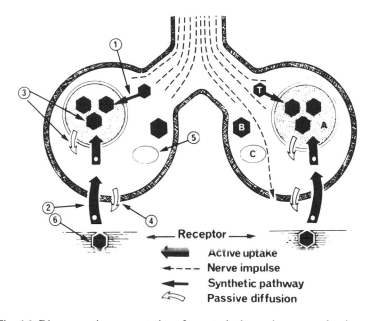

Fig. 6.1 Diagrammatic representation of a central adrenergic synapse showing possible sites of drug action. Right: A, granular pool of catecholamine; B, cytoplasmic pool of catecholamine; C, monoamine oxidase; T, precursors of catecholamines (tyrosine, etc.). Left: 1–6 see text.

in central tryptaminergic terminals and this has been used as a supplementary treatment for depression.

By blocking reuptake (Site 2). Monoamines are taken up again into nerve terminals after they have been released by an impulse, and are transported back into the granular stores ready for subsequent release. A drug preventing this reuptake will bring about an increase in the extraneuronal concentrations of noradrenaline and 5HT. This mechanism is thought to explain the therapeutic effects of the tricyclic antidepressants.

By modifying storage (Site 3). Reserpine and a related compound, tetrabenazine, block the uptake of monoamines into the granular stores, as well as promoting their release from these stores. The granules thus become depleted and this impairs transmission. The released transmitter is deaminated by MAO before leaving the terminals, and no initial stimulant effect is seen. Depletion of noradrenaline, dopamine and 5HT results in sedation and reduced motor activity, and suicidal depression has occurred with higher doses of reserpine in hypertensive patients. The depletion of dopamine from the corpus striatum can lead to Parkinsonism, but is turned to therapeutic use in the treatment of dyskinesias.

By promoting release from the terminals (Site 4). Some drugs, for example amphetamine, ephedrine and tyramine, are able to release monoamines from the nerve terminals in a physiologically-active form, mimicking transmission. They do not, however, deplete the granular stores to produce subsequent block.

By modifying breakdown (Site 5). The most important enzyme concerned in the breakdown of monoamines is MAO, which is situated in the nerve terminals. Inhibition of this enzyme leads to accumulation of monoamines, which in turn brings about an elevation in mood. MAO which is situated in the CNS differs from the peripheral enzyme and is called MAO-B. It can be selectively inhibited (p. 87).

By blocking postsynaptic receptors (Site 6). Phenothiazine compounds have, to varying extents, both α-adrenoceptor and dopamine-receptor blocking activity, which is partly responsible for their effects on behaviour and motor activity. The butyrophenones have dopamine blocking effects, but only exhibit α-blocking actions in high doses. Both groups of compound frequently produce Parkinsonism when prescribed in high dosage. Cyproheptadine is used as an antihistamine, but can also block 5HT receptors in the CNS.

By stimulating receptors (Site 6). Bromocriptine probably produces its effects by direct stimulation of dopamine receptors in the CNS (p. 87). It is believed that both opiates and benzodiazepines stimulate specific receptors in the CNS to produce their pharmacological effects.

DRUGS IN NEUROLOGY

Parkinsonism

Belladonna alkaloids were first used in the treatment of Parkinsonism just over 100 years ago, and anticholinergic drugs were the standard treatment until the 1960s, when further advances in therapy were stimulated by the observation that the concentration of dopamine in the corpus striatum of patients with idiopathic and postencephalitic Parkinsonism is reduced. Subsequently levodopa was administered to a few patients and encouraging results were obtained. This substance has emerged from innumerable clinical trials as the drug of choice in Parkinsonism.

The evidence for a regulatory mechanism in the striatum which is set by antagonistic effects of two transmitters, acetylcholine and dopamine, is now substantial, but the main points are as follows:

(a) Parkinsonism is alleviated by drugs which increase striatal dopamine or block the actions of acetylcholine.

(b) Drugs which deplete dopamine stores, e.g. reserpine, or block dopamine receptors, e.g. chlorpromazine, can induce or exacerbate Parkinsonism.

(c) Similarly, cholinomimetic or anticholinesterase drugs which penetrate into the brain, e.g. pilocarpine or physostigmine, worsen pre-existing disease.

(d) In experimental animals application of acetylcholine or carbachol to the caudate nucleus produces tremor and rigidity, which can be reversed by atropine or dopamine.

(e) Application of acetylcholine to single caudate neurones excites them, while dopamine usually inhibits them.

(f) The presence of high concentrations of acetylcholine, dopamine and the enzymes concerned in their synthesis and degradation have been demonstrated in the corpus striatum of animals and man.

The nerve terminals in the striatum which contain dopamine belong to a pathway from the substantia nigra, the nigro-striate pathway. Experimental lesions of these fibres in the monkey deplete striatal dopamine and produce contralateral hypokinesia and tremor. In patients with idiopathic and post-encephalitic Parkinsonism neuropathological studies have demonstrated a selective degeneration of this pathway, and examination of the CSF has shown low levels of homovanillic acid, the chief breakdown product of dopamine. The integrity of the cholinergic fibres terminating in the striatum appear to be unchanged, and normal concentrations of the enzymes concerned with the synthesis and breakdown of acetylcholine have been demonstrated.

All the evidence, therefore, points to a regulatory system in which acetylcholine is excitatory and dopamine is inhibitory to nerve cells concerned in extrapyramidal control, and that a disturbance of the balance of this system, in favour of acetylcholine, produces the clinical signs of Parkinsonism. A proposed scheme is illustrated in Figure 6.2. The treatment of the disease is directed to restoring the balance.

Anticholinergic drugs

A large number of naturally-occurring or synthetic anticholinergic

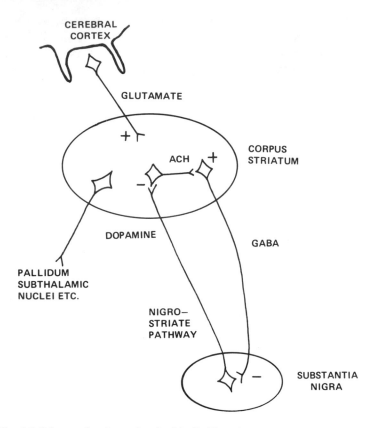

Fig. 6.2 Scheme of pathways involved in Parkinsonism.

drugs have been used in the treatment of Parkinsonism. Many of these have antihistamine properties in addition, but there is no evidence that this property is important. The more recent synthetic drugs do not seem to be superior to the more traditional compounds. Only limited improvement is seen, rigidity responding best, tremor less well, and hypokinesia little, if at all. The aetiology of the disease does not influence the response, and neither does treatment modify its course. It may be necessary to try different combinations of drugs, gradually increasing to maximum dosage, before an adequate response is seen.

Benzhexol is one of the most satisfactory and popular of these drugs, and has moderate potency. Benztropine is a more powerful drug, and can be useful given parenterally in the treatment of phenothiazine-induced dyskinesias. Orphenadrine is a less powerful anticholinergic, produces fewer side-effects, and is said to have a euphoriant action which makes it the drug of choice in depressed patients. This may be explained by its ability to block reuptake of dopamine and other monoamines into nerve terminals. Other drugs include procyclidine, methixene, and biperiden.

The side-effects of these drugs are predictable from their pharmacological actions. Parasympathetic blockade produces dry mouth, impairment of accommodation, constipation and hesitancy of micturition. Narrow angle glaucoma can be precipitated, and urinary retention can occur in males with prostatic hypertrophy. Confusion and hallucinations are seen in 20 to 30% of patients receiving the more powerful anticholinergics, and should be treated by withdrawal of the drug, and, if necessary, administration of an anticholinesterase which gains access to the brain, e.g. physostigmine.

Levodopa

Dopamine does not penetrate into the brain, so striatal dopamine levels can be increased only by giving its precursor, L-dopa, which is converted to the transmitter by the enzyme dopa decarboxylase.

The introduction of this drug represented a major advance in the treatment of a common and disabling disease. About one third of patients obtain very considerable benefit, the improvement occasionally being dramatic. Another third gain useful benefit, while the remainder are not helped or suffer disabling adverse effects. Idiopathic Parkinsonism shows the best response. Patients with postencephalitic disease tolerate levodopa poorly, often developing adverse effects with low doses. It is usually ineffective in patients with drug-induced Parkinsonism.

In contrast with anticholinergic drugs, levodopa usually produces considerable improvement in hypokinesia, which is one of the more disabling features of the disease. There is renewed ability to perform movements which have been lost for several years, and marked changes are seen in facial movements, walking, writing and speech. Rigidity is often reduced, but tremor is less consistently improved, and sometimes requires prolonged treatment before much change is seen. Previous treatment with anticholinergic drugs should be continued, as they have synergistic effects with levodopa, but phenothiazines, butyrophenones and reserpine should be stopped because they block the therapeutic effect. Pyridoxine (vitamin B_6) should not be given during levodopa treatment because it is converted into pyridoxal phosphate which forms a coenzyme to dopa decarboxylase, enhancing the peripheral decarboxylation of the drug. Thus, less is available to enter the brain. Many vitamin mixtures and tonics contain pyridoxine, and patients should be warned of this. Levodopa should never be given to patients receiving a conventional MAOI, for hypertensive crises can be provoked by doses as small as 50 mg but the selective MAO-B inhibitor, selegiline, is safe in this respect (see below).

Only a small fraction of the dose of levodopa reaches the corpus striatum and is converted into dopamine. The remainder is decarboxylated elsewhere, mainly peripherally.

This conversion at the other sites gives rise to adverse effects such as nausea and vomiting (an effect on dopamine receptors in the chemoreceptor trigger zone (CTZ) of the medulla), postural hypotension (by a central action and, possibly, by acting as a false transmitter peripherally), and psychiatric disturbances (by an effect on the mesolimbic system of the brain). Excessive dopaminergic stimulation in the striatum can lead to dyskinesias, particularly in patients with postencephalitic Parkinsonism.

These adverse effects are often dose-limiting when levodopa is given on its own. However, it is now usual to give a peripheral dopa decarboxylase inhibitor simultaneously with levodopa. Two combination preparations are available, Sinemet (which contains carbidopa as the peripheral dopa decarboxylase inhibitor) and Madopar (which contains benserazide). The inhibitors cannot penetrate into the brain, and therefore block the peripheral utilization of levodopa without affecting central metabolism. This has the advantage of reducing the dose of levodopa to about one quarter, mainly as a result of increased bioavailability by less first-pass metabolism, and lowering the incidence of nausea and vomiting. The reason for the latter is that the peripheral dopa decarboxylase inhibitors can gain access to the CTZ because the blood-brain barrier at this site is more permeable than elsewhere in the brain. The decarboxylation of levodopa is therefore prevented and the emetic effect of the drug, which is mediated via dopamine receptors in the CTZ, is reduced. However, nausea used to be dose-limiting when levodopa was given alone, and now that the therapeutic effect which can be achieved is greater in the absence of this limitation, the incidence of central adverse effects, such as dyskinetic reactions and psychiatric disturbances, are commoner. Dyskinesias occur as a result of excessive stimulation of dopamine receptors in the striatum; the characteristic features are lip-smacking and tongue protruding movements (bucco-lingual dyskinesia) but the neck, trunk and limbs may become involved if the dose is not reduced. Patients with postencephalitic Parkinsonism are more susceptible. Psychiatric disturbances comprise anxiety, restlessness, depression, confusion, delusions and sometimes frank psychosis; they result from excessive stimulation of mesolimbic dopamine receptors.

Levodopa is readily absorbed and produces peak plasma levels at 1–2 hours; it has a plasma half-life of about 3 hours. Although some of the adverse effects, e.g. nausea, coincide with this peak, the 'on-off' phenomenon (in which wide fluctuations in control are seen, sometimes over short periods of time) relates poorly to the pharmacokinetics of the drug although frequent small doses will often help. It occurs in patients with advanced disease.

Other adverse effects of levodopa include tachycardia and cardiac dysrhythmias, and a positive Coombs' test.

Amantadine

This was developed as an antiviral drug in influenza, but its anti-Parkinsonian effect was noticed in a clinical trial. It probably acts in an amphetamine-like manner, releasing catecholamines from nerve terminals. The clinical improvement induced by amantadine is much less than that produced by levodopa, but it is an easier drug to manage and the side-effects are fewer. Improvement is seen in all three major features, hypokinesia, rigidity and tremor. Drug-induced Parkinsonism does not respond.

The adverse effects of amantadine are dry mouth, defective near vision, constipation, confusion and hallucinations. A bluish-red skin discolouration, livideo reticularis, occurs in most patients, and ankle oedema is common.

Other drugs

Bromocriptine acts by directly stimulating the remaining dopamine receptors, but it has no advantages over levodopa plus a peripheral dopa decarboxylase inhibitor. It has similar adverse effects. It is used also in treating galactorrhoea and acromegaly (p. 204). Selegiline is a selective inhibitor of monoamine oxidase B, the enzyme variant that exists in the CNS. Given in conjunction with levodopa, it protects the dopamine which has been formed and is particularly useful in smoothing out the effect of levodopa in patients who experience dose-limiting adverse effects or the 'on-off' phenomenon. It does not inhibit MAO-A, the peripheral enzyme, and a hypertensive crisis is therefore not provoked by interaction with levodopa, as happens with conventional MAOIs.

Dyskinesia

Disturbance of extrapyramidal function can produce a number of syndromes in which involuntary movements predominate. The effectiveness of reserpine in Huntington's chorea was noted some years ago, but the drug produced many side-effects, particularly depression. Tetrabenazine is a drug with similar pharmacological actions, and is easier to manage. Trials have shown it to be effective in Huntington's chorea, other choreiform syndromes, dystonia and hemiballismus. These drugs produce their effects in these patients by depleting monoamines; patients dying with Huntington's chorea have an increase in dopamine concentration in the corpus striatum and pars compacta of the substantia nigra, as well as in the nucleus accumbens, and tetrabenazine probably works by depleting this transmitter.

Phenothiazines can also reduce abnormal movements, presumably by virtue of their blocking effects at central monoaminergic receptors. Thiopropazate, a piperazine derivative, seems to be of particular value in this respect.

Drug-induced extrapyramidal syndromes

The relationship between central catecholamine metabolism and extrapyramidal syndromes is a complex one. Depletion of the stores in nerve terminals with reserpine produces Parkinsonism, while increasing the concentration of catecholamines with levodopa leads to dyskinesia. Between these two extremes is a spectrum of disorders, most of which can be produced at various times by the phenothiazines. Acute dystonic reactions tend to occur in young patients, akathisia (motor restlessness) and tasikinesia (an inability to remain seated) in the middle aged, while Parkinsonism is the most common syndrome in the elderly. These reactions are usually reversible on stopping the offending drug. In contrast, irreversible tardive (i.e. late onset) dyskinesias can be produced by phenothiazines, and occur much more frequently than is generally realised, possibly in up to 25% of institutionalized patients. The complexity of these reactions is further illustrated by the fact the phenothiazines which produce dyskinesias can sometimes be useful for treating them.

Drug-induced Parkinsonism is little improved by levodopa or

amantadine. Where withdrawal of the offending drug is not possible, as is usually the case in schizophrenia, addition of an anticholinergic drug is helpful.

Levodopa-induced dyskinesia is almost invariably reversible,
unlike its phenothiazine counterpart. Although it can be effectively
treated with tetrabenazine or thiopropazate, these drugs also reverse
the anti-Parkinsonian action, so it is more rational to reduce the
dose of levodopa.

Epilepsy

Epileptic seizures are commonly caused by focal damage to the
brain as a result of a variety of physical insults. The seizures that
arise from these foci are called partial seizures, but they may progress to a tonic-clonic seizure by a process called secondary gener-
alization. In some patients, however, there is no evidence of focal
damage and the seizures are termed primary generalized or
idiopathic; they may be tonic-clonic in type (grand mal) or absences
(petit mal). Myoclonus may also be caused by a primary generalized
discharge.

The biochemical basis of epilepsy is poorly understood although
there is some evidence that GABA receptors are reduced in number
in epileptic foci. Furthermore, there is growing evidence that
several drugs which are used in treating seizures increase GABA
transmission. Experimental compounds that inhibit L-glutamate
decarboxylase (GAD) alter the balance between glutamate and
GABA in favour of the former, and this leads to the development
of seizures. On the other hand, drugs that inhibit GABA-glutamate
transaminase (GABA-T) inhibit seizures. It was thought that
sodium valproate acted in this way, but other mechanisms of action
are now thought to be more important. However, several potent
GABA-T inhibitors have been developed and preliminary trials look
promising.

GABA receptor agonists are also anticonvulsant although none
is yet available for clinical use. However, it is believed that benzodiazepine drugs, barbiturates and hydantoins enhance GABA transmission and this may account for their anticonvulsant activity.

In partial and tonic-clonic seizures, hydantoins, barbiturates,
carbamazepine and sodium valproate are used. Ethosuximide and
sodium valproate suppress petit mal absences, but the former drug
has no action against tonic-clonic seizures. Benzodiazepines are
useful both in status epilepticus and myoclonic seizures.

Hydantoins

These include phenytoin (diphenylhydantoin) and ethotoin. The first of these is the most widely used drug. It is hydroxylated in the liver by an enzyme system which is saturable, and in some patients up to 20 days may be required for the serum level to stabilize after changing the dose. The rate of metabolism of the drug varies greatly between patients, and one may be intoxicated by a dose which is therapeutically ineffective in another. Because of this it is necessary to increase the dose gradually until fit control is achieved or until signs of intoxication occur. The triad of signs which indicate over-dosage are nystagmus, ataxia, and dysarthria, signs of deranged cerebellar and brain stem function. If these signs are ignored permanent damage can result. Because of these uncertainties estimation of the serum level of the drug is invaluable. The aim is to produce a serum level of 40 to 80 μmol/l (10–20 μg/ml). The relationship between dose and serum level is a non-linear one, typical of saturation kinetics, and therefore increments in dose should become progressively smaller as the therapeutic range is reached (Fig. 6.3). Phenytoin has a long plasma half-life (30–60 hours) and therefore once-daily dosage gives stable control in adults, although twice-daily administration is preferable in children, who metabolize drugs more quickly.

Although phenytoin lacks the sedative property of phenobarbitone, it produces a greater variety of adverse reactions (see below).

Phenytoin is effective in suppressing tonic-clonic seizures, or the spread of a partial fit to a generalized one, but it is less valuable in suppressing the focus itself. It is of no value in absence seizures. Phenytoin has diverse pharmacological actions, including a direct depressant effect on the excitable membrane, enhancement of potassium transport into nerve cells, and potentiation of GABA transmission in the CNS. Which, if any, accounts for its anticonvulsant effect is not known. It also has a membrane stabilizing effect on the myocardium, and is a useful antidysrhythmic drug (p. 150).

Ethotoin is much less effective than phenytoin, although it is also less toxic.

Carbamazepine

Although related to the tricyclic antidepressants, carbamazepine is an effective anticonvulsant in tonic-clonic and partial seizures. It

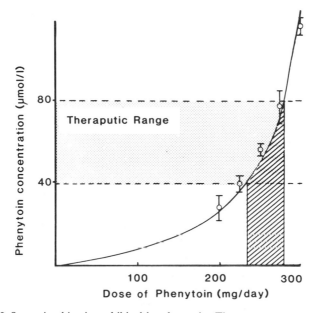

Fig. 6.3 Saturation kinetics exhibited by phenytoin. The measurements were obtained from one patient on several maintenance doses of phenytoin, and show a curvilinear relationship with a small dose range compatible with a therapeutic serum concerntration.

is probably as effective as phenytoin and phenobarbitone in tonic-clonic fits and may be superior to these two in partial epilepsies, in which it is regarded as a drug of first choice. It is to be preferred to barbiturates because it is less sedative, although dizziness is a common adverse effect. A psychotropic action has been claimed but this may simply reflect the lack of sedative effects compared with other anti-epileptic drugs rather than a direct pharmacological action.

Initially, carbamazepine acquired the reputation of being toxic on the bone marrow. Further experience has shown that, although rare cases of fatal agranulocytosis have been reported, the drug is remarkably safe in the epileptic patient. Bone marrow toxicity appears to be more common when the drug is used in trigeminal neuralgia, perhaps because of the greater age of patients with this condition.

Carbamazepine has a shorter plasma half-life than phenytoin, about 10–30 hours. It is particularly short in patients receiving combination therapy (its metabolism is inducible) and therefore it needs to be given two or three times daily. It is a potent liver enzyme inducing drug itself, and can therefore induce its own metabolism as well as that of other drugs. Its major metabolite is an epoxide, which also possesses antiepileptic activity, although somewhat less than the parent compound, and its plasma concentration in steady state is much lower.

Barbiturates

The introduction of phenobarbitone in 1912 provided the first potent anticonvulsant drug for the treatment of epilepsy. Only the long-acting barbiturates, e.g. barbitone, phenobarbitone and methylphenobarbitone, have useful anticonvulsant properties for oral treatment of chronic epilepsy. Some of the short-acting compounds actually have convulsant properties, and are used for activating although they can, paradoxically, be of value in the treatment of status (see below). Phenobarbitone is the most widely used barbiturate. It is metabolized slowly in the liver to hydroxyphenobarbitone but about 30% is excreted unchanged in the urine. It has a plasma half-life of 50–160 hours in the adult and therefore it is cumulative and takes about 30 days to reach a constant serum level. Hasty changes of treatment should not, therefore, be made, and 3 months or more may be required to assess the value of the drug adequately in any one patient. The drug should be given in one dose at night.

Sedation is one of the chief drawbacks of phenobarbitone, and often limits the dose. It is worse during the period when the dose is being built up, but tends to settle when a steady dose is arrived at. This is the result of tolerance, and withdrawal symptoms can occur after stopping the drug. These withdrawal symptoms include epileptic fits, and therefore reductions in dose should be made very gradually. Sudden withdrawal of phenobarbitone can precipitate status epilepticus. Phenobarbitone is poorly tolerated in children, causing impairment of learning capacity, irritability and disturbances of behaviour. If it is necessary to give a drug for tonic-clonic seizures to a child it is better to choose carbamazepine or sodium valproate.

These adverse effects make phenobarbitone no longer a drug of first choice and it should be used only when phenytoin or carbamazepine have been ineffective. The mode of action of the anticonvulsant barbiturates is uncertain, although there is evidence that they enhance GABA transmission.

Primidone is structurally closely related to the barbiturates and is, in fact, oxidized partly into phenobarbitone by liver enzymes. For this reason combinations of phenobarbitone and primidone should be avoided. Some patients are intolerant of primidone, and an initial test dose of a quarter of a tablet is advisable. Blood dyscrasias are more common with this drug than with phenobarbitone.

Sodium valproate

This compound is structurally very different from any other anti-epileptic drug, being a simple two chain fatty acid. It inhibits GABA-glutamate transaminase and succinic semialdehyde dehydrogenase, enzymes which are responsible for GABA metabolism in the brain, which may partly account for its anti-epileptic effects. However, it also has a direct effect on the permeability of the neuronal membrane It has a broad spectrum of action, and it is a drug of first choice in both absence and myoclonic seizures. It has an advantage over ethosuximide for these types of seizures in that it is also active against co-existing tonic clonic fits. In partial seizures it is less impressive.

It is relatively free from adverse effects, but will potentiate the sedative effects of phenobarbitone and primidone by inhibiting their metabolism. Increased appetite, tremor and reversible hair loss occur occasionally and hepatotoxicity has been reported, rarely fatal. It has a short half-life (8–15 hours), but, paradoxically, it has a long duration of action (a 'hit-and-run' type of action) and once or twice daily dosage appears to be satisfactory. The drug circulates in plasma as valproic acid, which is over 90% bound to plasma proteins. It is displaced by free fatty acids and spontaneous fluctuation of their concentration in plasma causes variation in the binding, and therefore the plasma concentration of valproic acid.

Ethosuximide

Ethosuximide is a succinimide compound that is used for the treatment of absences and myoclonic seizures. In tonic-clonic and partial seizures it is ineffective. It can be combined with any of those for major epilepsy when both types of fit coexist but single drug treatment with sodium valproate is preferable in these circumstances. Ethosuximide has a long plasma half-life (20–40 hours in children) and once or twice daily dosage is satisfactory.

Toxic effects include nausea and vomiting, dizziness and drowsiness, and leucopenia.

Oxazolidinediones

Paramethadione and trimethadione (troxidone) were the predecessors to ethosuximide. They are now infrequently used because they are less effective than ethosuximide and are more toxic. Adverse effects include glare phenomenon and photobia, skin rashes, blood dyscrasias and hepatic and renal damage.

Benzodiazepines

The benzodiazepine drugs are widely used for treating status epilepticus (see below) although their long-term oral use in epilepsy has been disappointing, because central tolerance occurs. The most potent anticonvulsant 1, 4-benzodiazepine, clonazepam, is effective in absences and myoclonic seizures, but is very sedative. Sodium valproate should always be tried first. Nitrazepam has been widely used in massive infantile spasms (salaam spasms, hypsarrhythmia). It causes hypersalivation in large doses. Clobazam, a 1, 5-benzodiazepine, also has good anticonvulsant activity, and it tends to produce euphoria rather than sedation.

Other anticonvulsants

Sulthiame, a sulphonamide derivative, is used less now than in the past. It is active against partial and tonic-clonic seizures, but it has the major disadvantage of inhibiting the metabolism of other antiepileptic drugs. It can cause parasthesiae and hyperpnoea. Beclamide, a drug which is said to have stimulant rather than sedative properties, is only a weak anticonvulsant and is little used. Acetazolamide, the carbonic anhydrase inhibitor and diuretic, has been used in petit mal absences, but its effect is not impressive. ACTH and corticosteroids are often helpful in infantile spasms, although they do not influence the long-term prognosis.

Adverse effects of anti-epileptic drug therapy

All of the available anti-epileptic drugs have a narrow therapeutic ratio and therefore dose-related adverse effects are common, such as nystagmus, ataxia and dysarthria caused by phenytoin, sedation due to phenobarbitone and primidone, and dizziness and double vision with carbamazepine.

With long-term use, other problems arise. Phenytoin causes an unusual adverse effect, gum hyperplasia. Although it is dose related, its severity varies considerably from one patient to another. Coarse features and hirsutes can also be caused by this drug. Behavioural disturbances and impairment of learning ability are common, particularly with phenobarbitone, primidone and phenytoin. Paradoxical irritability and hyperkinesia may occur in young children.

Phenytoin, phenobarbitone, primidone and carbamazepine (but not sodium valproate or benzodiazepines) induce hepatic microsomal enzymes. This causes induction of the metabolism of other anti-epileptic drugs, resulting in low plasma levels with multiple drug therapy. It also reduces the effectiveness of other drugs which are metabolized in the liver, such as oral anticoagulants, the combined contraceptive pill and corticosteroid drugs. The metabolism of endogenous substances may also be disturbed, such as folic acid (occasionally leading to red cell macrocytosis), vitamin D (causing osteomalacia) and steroid hormones.

The incidence of congenital malformations in the offspring of epileptic women is 2–3 times greater than normal. This is probably in part due to anti-epileptic drug therapy, although genetic factors may also contribute. Hare lip and cleft palate, and cardiovascular anomalies are particularly common. The relative teratogenic potencies of the individual drugs has not been elucidated. Sodium valproate is thought to increase the incidence of spina bifida. In addition to teratogenic effects, anti-epileptic drugs can cause a bleeding tendency at birth because the production of clotting factors in the neonate is disturbed. Anti-epileptic drugs are lipid soluble and therefore appear in breast milk, but the total dose received by the baby is generally insufficient to make breast feeding indesirable.

Drugs for status epilepticus

Fits are potentially damaging to the brain. This applies particularly to status in childhood, which can lead to permanent temporal lobe damage, and this can in turn result in temporal lobe epilepsy. Status is therefore an emergency and should be terminated as quickly as possible. Diazepam given intravenously is regarded as the drug of choice although other benzodiazepine drugs such as clonazepam or lorazepam may be equally effective. Sometimes the effect of diazepam is only transient, and it may have to be given in repeated doses. Infusion over long periods should be avoided, however, because prolonged coma can result from accumulation of N-desmethyldiazepam, which is only slowly eliminated (p. 124). Diazepam causes significant respiratory depresion and hypotension only when other drugs, e.g. phenobarbitone, have been given parenterally before it. Intravenous phenytoin is an alternative, given as a loading dose of 15 mg/kg (assuming the patient has not been on chronic phenytoin therapy) followed by a daily maintenance dose. Intramuscularly, phenytoin is highly irritant and badly absorbed. Phenobarbitone is unsatisfactory in status because it penetrates the blood-brain barrier only slowly. If diazepam is used initially to stop the acute episode, phenytoin or phenobarbitone should subsequently be administered parenterally to prevent recurrence. Chlormethiazole given by intravenous infusion is very effective and the drug has the advantage of a short plasma half-life. It frequently causes thrombophlebitis. Thiopentone, or some other short-acting barbiturate, given as an initial intravenous injection may be effective, but infusion should be avoided because the elimination half-life of the drug is long (unlike the distribution half-life which determines the duration of unconsciousness after a single dose) and, like diazepam, prolonged coma can result. Paraldehyde given intramuscularly, or slowly intravenously after dilution, is still used by some. It is relatively safe, although it has a number of disadvantages.

Occasionally status may be resistant to one or several of the above drugs. It may then be necessary to anaesthetise and curarize the patient and maintain breathing by intermittent positive pressure ventilation through a tracheostomy tube.

Drugs which can cause fits

It is important to bear in mind the potential convulsant action of some drugs, for they should not, if possible, be given to epileptic patients, and they may occasionally precipitate a fit in a patient who has never previously had one. Drugs possessing this action include the phenothiazines, tricyclic and tetracyclic antidepressants, aminophylline and many antihistamines. Abrupt withdrawal of barbiturates or benzodiazepines can also precipitate fits. Drugs given intrathecally, especially penicillin and antimitotic drugs readily produce fits.

Narcolepsy

This is a rare condition which includes an uncontrollable desire to sleep, hypnogogic hallucinations, and sleep paralysis. Amphetamine is the best treatment but the tricyclic antidepressants, particularly clomipramine, are effective when cataplexy is prominent.

Migraine

The aetiology of migraine is disputed. Most theories have centred around a vascular origin for the pain, resulting from a dilatation of cranial vessels. Several chemical theories have been put forward to explain this dilatation, including a change in levels of circulating histamine, acetylcholine, 5HT and, most recently, prostaglandins. An alternative explanation is that migraine arises in the brain stem as a paroxysmal sympathetic discharge. The demonstration of a reduced venous 5HT level in migraine, and the prophylactic value of methysergide, a potent 5HT antagonist, have lent support to the view that this monoamine is involved in the genesis of migraine attacks, but the results of the 5HT measurements require corroboration. A defect in tyramine metabolism has been suggested, and would explain the association between various foods and migraine attacks in some patients. The high incidence of non-specific EEG abnormalities have led some to postulate a cerebral cause for the attacks, and phenytoin has been claimed to be of value in treatment. Because of these uncertainties about the aetiology of the disease, there is no logical treatment. Nausea and gastric stasis may occur early in a migraine attack, reducing the absorption of analgesic drugs given by the oral route. Metoclopramide, administered parenterally or rectally, may increase the rate of gastric emptying and so improve the absorption of analgesic drugs from the gastrointestinal tract. Traditional antiemetics such as cyclizine or prochlorperazine are less useful because their anticholinergic effects may adversely affect gastrointestinal motility.

Mild analgesics

These should be tried first, for they benefit a substantial proportion of patients, and have fewer side-effects. Aspirin and paracetamol are satisfactory. Soluble and effervescent preparations act more quickly.

Ergotamine tartrate

This is frequently of value in classical migraine when taken at the first warning of an attack. It is valueless if it is taken when the attack is established. In addition to its α-adrenolytic action, ergotamine has a direct constrictor effect on vascular smooth muscle, reversing the dilatation of cranial vessels.

The drug can be given in a variety of ways and forms. Intramuscular injection is probably the most satisfactory, but is often impractical. Inhalation by aerosol (Medihaler–ergotamine) is rapidly effective. The drug is absorbed from the buccal mucous membrane, and sublingual tablets (Lingraine) or tablets for chewing (Cafergot-Q) are useful. Oral administration is the most popular, although the drug is absorbed less rapidly. Absorption appears to be increased by addition of caffeine, which a number of proprietary preparations contain. The content of ergotamine varies from 1 to 2 mg, but no more than 12 mg should be taken in a week. Overdosage can cause peripheral vasoconstriction (St. Anthony's fire), gangrene of the extremities and headaches which may mimic the migraine syndrome which is being treated. Ergot-containing drugs should be avoided in pregnancy and cardiovascular disease. They should not be used for prophylaxis in migraine, although in cluster headaches it may be helpful.

Dihydroergotamine less frequently produces side-effects, but is also less effective.

Prophylactic drugs

Propranolol is often helpful in reducing the frequency of migraine attacks. It is of interest in this respect that it has serotonin antagonist effects in addition to its β-blocking activity. It should not be given with ergotamine because they both increase peripheral resistance.

Pizotifen is structurally similar to cyproheptadine and the tricyclic antidepressants, and is a serotonin antagonist. It is often effective in prophylaxis but drowsiness and weight gain are common.

Another serotonin antagonist, methysergide, is an effective drug in preventing attacks, but its chief disadvantage is the frequency, and occasional severity, of adverse effects. Nausea, drowsiness and unsteadiness are common, and peripheral vasoconstriction occurs, producing numbness, parasthesiae and muscle cramps. Perceptual changes and hallucinations have been seen. But the most serious complication is retroperitoneal fibrosis, leading to hydronephrosis. Fibrosis in pleural and pericardial cavities also occurs.

Clonidine (p. 72) reduces the responsiveness of peripheral

vessels to both dilator and constrictor effects of catecholamines, which may account for its effectiveness as a prophylactic drug in migraine. It is given in much smaller doses than for hypertension, and with these doses adverse effects are few.

Trigeminal neuralgia

Injection of alcohol or phenol into the gasserian ganglion, as was once the standard treatment for trigeminal neuralgia, has now been made obsolete by an effective drug, carbamazepine, which was introduced initially for epilepsy (p. 90). Whether trigeminal neuralgia is caused by an 'epileptiform' discharge somewhere along the trigeminal sensory pathway is disputed. Other anticonvulsant drugs, e.g. phenytoin, have also been used, but are less effective.

Bell's palsy

Although the cause of this condition is not known, there is evidence that ACTH and steroids reduce the incidence and lessen the severity of denervation when given in high dosage as soon after the onset of symptoms as possible. Steroids may be preferable to ACTH.

Spasticity

In spasticity there is an increase in the excitability either of spinal α-motoneurones or of fusimotor neurones; sometimes both are hyperactive. This is caused by an imbalance of descending excitatory and inhibitory tone resulting from a lesion of the corticospinal pathway, although the nature of the change in transmitter action is unknown. However, this abnormal state of affairs can be reversed either by reducing descending facilitation from the brain stem, or by a direct action on synaptic transmission in the spinal cord. Several tranquillizers have actions at both levels, but the relative importance of these mechanisms in producing the muscle relaxant effect of these drugs is uncertain. None of them is entirely satisfactory, for sedation often becomes a problem before much relief from spasticity has been achieved.

Diazepam (p. 122) is one of the more effective compounds for treating spasticity, and probably works mainly by facilitating GABA transmission in the spinal cord. GABA is known to act as a transmitter mediating presynaptic inhibition in the spinal cord.

Diazepam is the most active of the benzodiazepines on muscle tone. Occasionally, extensor hypotonus can occur, making walking so difficult that treatment has to be discontinued.

Baclofen is a derivative of GABA, which probably acts as a general neuronal depressant in the spinal cord rather than by mimicking GABA. It is a drug of first choice in spasticity, but frequently produces nausea, dizziness and hypotension.

Dantrolene is a hydantoin which impairs excitation contraction coupling in skeletal muscle, and appears to be useful in spasticity. It commonly causes muscle weakness, light headedness and diarrhoea.

Methocarbamol and chlormezanone are of little practical value although they continue to be marketed for muscle spasm associated with minor sprains and injuries. Quinine is used for relieving nocturnal leg cramps.

Neuromuscular junction

Neuromuscular blocking drugs

The neuromuscular junction can be blocked in one of two ways, (a) by competitive inhibition, whereby the blocking drug antagonizes acetylcholine in proportion to its concentration at the receptor site, and (b) by depolarization of the end plate beyond the threshold required to generate an action potential in the muscle fibre. As the triggering threshold is passed an action potential may be produced, accounting for the initial muscle twitching which depolarizing drugs produce. This often causes subsequent aching in the muscles resulting from slight damage produced by incoordinated contractions. The competitive antagonists do not have this effect, and they can prevent the twitching from depolarizing drugs when given in small dosage just before administration of the depolarizer. The depolarizing drugs also produce a degree of desensitization of the receptors to acetylcholine, and this may in part account for their blocking action. Competitive blockade can be reversed by an anticholinesterase drug, which prevents breakdown of the transmitter and leads to its accumulation at the receptor site, changing the balance of concentrations in favour of acetycholine. Anticholinesterases deepen, rather than reverse, a depolarizing block, for accumulation of acetylcholine produces further depolarization. In fact, anticholinesterases in sufficient doses can themselves produce muscle fasciculation and depolarizing block.

Tubocurarine and gallamine are both competitive drugs. Up to 3 minutes is required for maximum effect after injection. The action of gallamine lasts for 20 to 30 minutes, while tubocurarine has a slightly longer action. Gallamine can cause tachycardia from vagal inhibition, and tubocurarine produces slight hypotension from ganglionic blockade, and occasional histamine release producing flushing of the skin of the head and neck.

Pancuronium, another competitive blocker, has replaced tubocurarine for major surgery, and has a quicker onset of action. It does not cause histamine release or lower the blood pressure. Alcuronium and vecuronium are similar to tubocurarine. Fazidinium has the most rapid onset of action and acts for about 40 minutes. Atracurium is eliminated by a non-enzymatic reaction which is independent of hepatic and renal function.

Suxamethonium (succinyl choline) is the only useful depolarizing drug. It acts in 1 minute and its effects last for up to 5 minutes making it suitable for short anaesthetic procedures such as ECT. It has slight muscarinic effects, causing bradycardia from vagal stimulation. It should not be mixed with thiopentone is a syringe, for the alkalinity of the latter drug causes hydrolysis of suxamethonium. Plasma cholinesterase hydrolyses the drug to succinyl monocholine and finally succinic acid and choline, and enzyme variants can occasionally result in prolonged paralysis and apnoea. A pair of non-dominant autosomal genes determines the type of enzyme. Heterozygotes (3% of the population) may have slightly delayed recovery, while homozygotes for the atypical gene (0.03%) may take many hours to regain spontaneous breathing. Enzyme variants can be detected by measuring the degree to which the local anaesthetic, dibucaine, inhibits the enzyme.

Neuromuscular blocking drugs can be potentiated by aminoglycoside antibiotics, particularly neomycin, kanamycin and streptomycin, and by chlorpromazine and some general anaesthetic agents. Long-acting anticholinesterases used in the prophylactic treatment of glaucoma, can cause resistance to competitive antagonists. Patients with latent or overt myasthenia are particularly sensitive to neuromuscular blockade, and this has occasionally been used as a diagnostic test, but one which requires ventilation apparatus close to hand.

Anticholinesterases

These compounds impede the action of cholinesterase in one of two ways, either (1) by possessing a kationic group, usually a quaternary ammonium, which has affinity for the anionic site of the enzyme, thus preventing the union of enzyme and substrate; or (2) by acting as a false substrate, but one which forms an intermediate compound which can only by hydrolyzed slowly ('reversible') or not at all ('irreversible').

Edrophonium has the first type of action, while all the other commonly used drugs act as false substrates. Physostigmine, neostigmine and pyridostigmine form intermediate compounds which are hydrolyzed in a matter of hours, and the enzyme is released again for combination with acetyl choline, but the organophosphorus compounds produce stable intermediates, and new cholinesterase has to be synthesized, which may take up to several weeks to be complete.

Anticholinesterases have several clinical uses.

(a) Reversal of competitive neuromuscular blockade following surgery. Neostigmine remains the most useful drug for this purpose.

(b) Diagnosis of myasthenia gravis, or differential diagnosis between cholinergic crisis and myasthenic weakness (see below).

(c) Treatment of myasthenia gravis (see below).

(d) Treatment of paralytic ileus, bladder atony or supraventricular tachycardia. A drug with marked muscarinic effects, such as neostigmine, is required for this purpose.

(e) Treatment of glaucoma. Eye drops containing physostigmine, neostigmine or an organophosphorous compound can be used to keep the pupil constricted in narrow angle glaucoma.

Edrophonium has predominantly nicotinic effects, some of which are the result of direct stimulation of receptors in addition to its anticholinesterase activity, and it can cause muscle fasciculation in small doses or a depolarization block in larger doses. Its effects last for 10 minutes. Neostigmine has a longer duration of action, producing a useful effect for up to 4 hours or more. Its marked muscarinic effects are a disadvantage when the drug is being used for its neuromuscular actions, and often require addition of atropine or a similar drug to block muscarinic receptors. This is especially so when it is given to patients with myasthenia, when intestinal colic is frequently produced. Physostigmine is now obsolete clinically, except for its use in glaucoma. Pyridostigmine is a longer-acting preparation than neostigmine, and is used in treating myasthenia. Ambenonium, a quaternary ammonium compound, has a slightly longer duration of action, while distigmine has the longest duration of action of the whole group and may be cumulative when given regularly.

The organophosphorus compounds, e.g. dyflos, echothiophate and tetraethylpyrophosphate, have been developed primarily as insecticides or 'nerve gases', but are of value for long-term treatment of glaucoma, for which they are instilled into the eye in an oily vehicle once every few days. Unfortunately, they may cause anterior lens opacities and other ocular effects, and may be sufficiently absorbed systemically to produce resistance to competitive neuromuscular blockade, or even frank muscarinic effects. Poisoning with these compounds can be a serious matter, but the development of cholinesterase reactivators has provided an effective treatment. These drugs, e.g. pralidoxime (P2S), combine with the phosphorylated enzyme but have a greater affinity for the organophosphorus moiety, breaking its linkage with the enzyme. The reactivator must be given as soon as possible, certainly within a few hours, to be effective, for a chemical change in the organophosphorus-enzyme complex slowly takes place and a much more stable compound results.

Myasthenia gravis

In myasthenia gravis there is an impairment of transmission at the neuromuscular junction, and in some patients high titres of an antibody to the acetylcholine receptor can be found in plasma. Plasmaphoresis may help these patients, but the conventional therapy is with anticholinesterases. Treatment is aimed at increasing the concentration of free acetycholine at the junction, by inhibiting cholinesterase with anticholinesterase drugs, and this overcomes the deficient transmission. However, in excess, anticholinesterases can produce muscle fasciculation and depolarization block, and for each patient there is an optimum dose which produces maximum benefit without causing block, the so-called 'cholinergic crisis'. A patient with severe myasthenia usually has a lower plateau of response, and it is these patients in whom overdosage is most likely to occur. Sometimes it is impossible to distinguish between a worsening myasthenic state and a cholinergic crisis without resorting to a pharmacological test. Here the short duration of action of edrophonium is invaluable. An intravenous injection of 2 mg will produce prompt improvement when myasthenic weakness is the main problem, but will briefly worsen neuromuscular transmission in a cholinergic crisis. This test is also useful in the diagnosis of myasthenia gravis, which is the only form of muscle weakness which will respond to an anti-cholinesterase.

For regular maintenance therapy these drugs are given orally. Neostigmine is still widely used but its short duration of action (4 hours) and potent effect are disadvantages. Pyridostigmine may be preferable particularly when the patient is weak on awakening, and produces fewer unwanted muscarinic effects. Ambenonium and distigmine have an even longer duration of action but may accumulate and cause depolarization block.

Severe intoxication with anticholinesterase drugs, causing embarrassed breathing and swallowing, can be treated with an intravenous oxime cholinesterase reactivator, but this is seldom necessary. Temporary withdrawal of the drug is all that need be done in most cases. Unwanted muscarinic effects are frequently troublesome, particularly after the first dose of the day, but can be prevented by addition of atropine or a similar muscarinic blocking drug which may require parenteral administration because of gastrointestinal hurry.

Corticosteroids are of value in patients who derive little benefit from conventional therapy. Long-term improvement may occur although there may be transient initial worsening. Azathioprine may also be of value.

Several drugs are capable of causing or precipitating a myasthenic state in some patients. These include the aminoglycoside antibiotics streptomycin, neomycin and kanamycin, and phenytoin and phenothiazines.

ANTI-EMETICS

Central vomiting can be induced by stimulation either of the emetic centre in the brain stem, or of the chemoreceptor trigger zone (CTZ) situated in the floor of the fourth ventricle. Various centrally-acting emetic drugs act by stimulating the CTZ, but they will cause vomiting only when the emetic centre is intact, for it is the final common pathway for all emetic stimuli. Two classes of compound are useful anti-emetics, dopamine receptor antagonists and anti-cholinergic drugs. The former block emetic stimuli acting through the CTZ whereas the latter act directly on the emetic centre. Some antihistamines also have effective anti-emetic properties, but these are probably accounted for by the marked anticholinergic actions of these compounds. Some dopamine receptor antagonists such as the phenothiazines have atropine-like actions

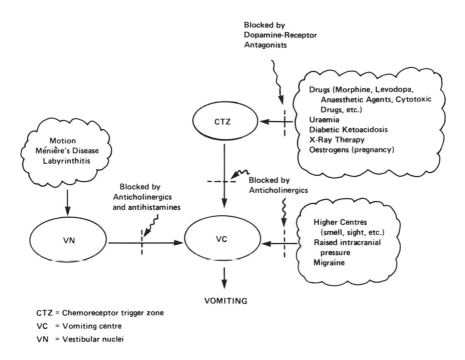

CTZ = Chemoreceptor trigger zone
VC = Vomiting centre
VN = Vestibular nuclei

Fig. 6.4 Stimuli which can produce central vomiting, and their blockade by anti-emetic drugs.

also, and they probably act on the emetic centre in addition to their effect on the CTZ. Figure 6.4 summarizes the various stimuli which can evoke central vomiting.

Anti-emetics acting on the CTZ

The phenothiazines which have been most widely used as anti-emetics are chlorpromazine, prochlorperazine, perphenazine, trifluoperazine and thiethylperazine. The first of these is the most sedative but there are no clear differences in efficacy. These drugs are discussed more fully on p. 118.

Metoclopramide is a dopamine receptor antagonist chemically related to procaine, but lacking local anaesthetic activity and possessing a market anti-emetic effect, a direct stimulant effect on gastric motility, possibly by sensitizing the smooth muscle to acetylcholine, and a weak antipsychotic action. The effect on gastric motility is particularly useful in speeding up radiological examination of the small intestine by contrast media, in facilitating duodenal intubation, in helping to prevent aspiration of gastric contents during emergency surgery, in promoting the absorption of oral analgesic drugs in migraine, and in relieving pyloric spasm and nausea associated with upper gastro-intestinal disease. It can cause acute dystonic reactions, particularly in children, as a result of its actions in the striatum; in this way it resembles the phenothiazines, particularly those with a piperazine structure (p. 118).

Domperidone is structurally unrelated but is similar in its actions to metoclopramide. It crosses the blood-brain barrier less readily and is therefore less likely to produce dystonic reactions. Cardiac dysrhythmias can occur following intravenous injection of the drug.

Nabilone is a synthetic cannabinoid which is particularly useful in treating the nausea caused by cytotoxic drugs and probably acts on the CTZ.

Drug-induced vomiting. A large number of drugs can induce central vomiting, but the most important are morphine and other narcotic drugs, cytotoxic drugs, oestrogens, dopaminergic agonists (e.g. levodopa, bromocriptine) and volatile anaesthetic agents. As these act on the CTZ it is logical to treat vomiting due to these agents with metoclopramide, domperidone or a phenothiazine.

Metabolic vomiting. The vomiting accompanying diabetic keto-acidosis, uraemia, or deep X-ray therapy can be counteracted by dopamine receptor antagonists, although anticholinergics are often equally effective.

Vomiting of pregnancy. Nausea and vomiting during the first trimester is very common and is probably related to the rapid rise in circulating oestrogens. It is preferable to avoid anti-emetic drugs if possible, but a phenothiazine, antihistamine or metoclopramide may be used it vomiting becomes frequent. Thiethylperazine suppositories may be of value. Dicyclomine is frequently used, although there has been some doubt about its teratogenic potential. Pyridoxine is included in some propriety preparations on the grounds that pyridoxine deficiency can cause vomiting, but there is no evidence that it is of any value.

Anti-emetics acting on the emetic centre

Where the emetic stimulus is directly on the emetic centre, e.g. by excessive vestibular stimulation in travel sickness or Ménière's disease, an anticholinergic drug should be chosen, such as hyoscine or an antihistamine or phenothiazine with anticholinergic actions.

Examples of antihistamines used in this situation are cinnarizine, cyclizine, dimenhydrinate, meclozine, mepyramine and promethazine (a phenothiazine antihistamine).

Motion sickness. Excessive vestibular stimulation can lead to vomiting, especially in children. In predisposed subjects anti-emetic drugs should be used prophylactically, taken 1 hour before starting the journey. Hyoscine, cyclizine and meclozine are the most popular, the first being the most powerful. Promethazine is also effective, but is more sedative. Dry mouth, blurred vision and sedation are common.

Ménière's disease. The vertigo and vomiting of this condition result from excessive stimulation of vestibular pathways by disease of the labyrinth. Anti-emetic drugs can be given prophylactically to reduce the severity of the attacks, but their effectiveness is difficult to assess. In prolonged attacks the sedative effects of prochlorperazine or promethazine may be of value, although as antiemetics they are not as effective as anticholinergics or antihistamines. Betahistine and cinnarizine have been promoted for Ménière's disease, and may be marginally more effective than other drugs.

Peripheral vomiting. Stimulation of autonomic afferent fibres from the thoracic and abdominal viscera can induce vomiting, e.g. following a myocardial infarction, from ingestion of a gastric irritant, or from peptic ulceration. Centrally-acting anti-emetics are of little value in these conditions. Sometimes, however, vomiting is caused partly by an opiate and partly by the condition for which it is being given, e.g. myocardial infarction, and in this case a phenothiazine anti-emetic will be of value.

Antispasmodics may be useful in some cases of peripheral vomiting. Dicyclomine, for instance, is effective in infantile vomiting and colic.

Emetic agents

The production of vomiting is occasionally of value, especially following a drug overdose. Simple measures, such as digital stimulation of the pharynx can be effective. Ipecacuanha induces vomiting partly by a central action and partly by a local irritant one. It is slow in its action, and this limits its usefulness in drug overdosage. It is contained in small amounts in some cough linctuses, and a purified form of it, emetine, is used as an amoebicide.

Apomorphine is a semisynthetic opiate with weak analgesic and strong emetic actions. It stimulates the CTZ. Given subcutaneously it induces vomiting within a few minutes, but is too potent for clinical use.

LOCAL ANAESTHETIC AGENTS

Many drugs have local anaesthetic properties, but the only ones which are clinically useful in this respect are those which do not, at the same time, cause tissue irritation. Local anaesthesia is the result of a block of transmission in nerve fibres or their associated sensory receptors. All types of nerve are affected although small fibres are blocked first, accounting for the dissociation of pain and touch which frequently occurs during onset of, or recovery from, anaesthesia. The blockade of transmission is caused by an inhibition of the sodium influx which occurs during a propagated spike potential. This effect occurs in all excitable tissues if the local concentration is high enough. Thus local anaesthetic drugs can have antidysrhythmic and anticonvulsant properties, which are of clinical value with lignocaine. Unfortunately, toxic effects on the central nervous system also occur, producing restlessness, tremor and even convulsions.

Cocaine

This is little used now, except for surface anaesthesia of the cornea and respiratory passages (during bronchoscopy), but it is no longer the most suitable drug for these purposes. It has sympathomimetic properties by blocking reuptake of noradrenaline into nerve terminals. In the eye it causes blanching of the sclera, mydriasis and a widening of the palpebral fissure. With frequent use it can cause desquamation and ulceration of the conjunctival epithelium. Despite its vasoconstricting properties, it is rapidly absorbed from mucous membranes and can readily produce toxic effects. It stimulates the highest centres of the brain, which accounts for its addiction potential. With chronic misuse it leads to delusions, hallucinations and paranoid ideas.

Procaine

Procaine is not suitable for surface use, for it is poorly absorbed from mucous membranes. When injected, it is rapidly hydrolysed by pseudocholinesterase in the serum, producing para-aminobenzoic acid. This substance can antagonize the bacteriostatic action of sulphonamides. It produces vasodilatation when infiltrated into tissues, and this shortens its duration of action.

Lignocaine

This is one of the most popular of local anaesthetics. It is rapidly absorbed from mucous surfaces and diffuses quickly into the tissues. When injected, it has a relatively short duration of action (30–60 minutes) but this can be prolonged by addition of adrenaline (see below). It is used for infiltration, regional nerve block and spinal anaesthesia, has little effect on blood vessel tone and is less toxic than procaine. It is metabolized in the liver, and not by pseudocholinesterase.

Bupivacaine

Bupivacaine has a slow onset of action when injected but produces prolonged anaesthesia, lasting up to 8 hours. It is particularly useful for epidural analgesia in obstetrics, and spinal anaesthesia.

Others

Prilocaine is similar to lignocaine, although less toxic, and is used in dentistry. Amethocaine is powerfully surface-active and is popular in ophthalmology. Its toxicity makes it unsuitable for injection. Cinchocaine is also toxic, but is is sometimes used for spinal anaesthesia. Benzocaine is relatively weak, but finds favour in a proprietary preparation promoted for sore throats.

Clinical use

In dentistry lignocaine containing 1:80 000–200 000 adrenaline is widely used. The sympathomimetic amine is added to produce vasoconstriction, making the resulting anaesthesia more reliable and of longer duration. It is preferable to avoid the use of adrenaline in patients with heart disease or hyperthyroidism, for the β-adrenergic stimulant actions of the amine can cause dysrhythmias. It should not be used in patients receiving treatment with a tricyclic antidepressant, for its pressor effects are potentiated. Felypressin, a polypeptide which produces vasoconstriction by a direct action on vascular smooth muscle, does not interact with tricyclic drugs. MAOIs do not potentiate direct acting sympathomimetic agents.

Local anaesthetics with vasoconstrictors are useful in medical work for suturing skin wounds or infiltrating the abdominal wall before incision during an operation under local anaesthesia. They should be assiduously avoided, however, for producing ring-block of an extremity, such as a finger, toe or pinna, for they can cause prolonged ischaemia which sometimes leads to gangrene of the part.

Further reading

Calne D B 1980 Therapeutics in neurology, 2nd ed. Blackwell, Oxford
Klawans H L, Weiner W J 1981 Textbook of clinical neuropharmacology. Raven Press, New York

7

Psychopharmacology

At the beginning of the previous chapter the current state of knowledge about transmitters in the CNS and their modification by drug therapy was outlined. The importance particularly of mono-aminergic transmission, i.e. utilizing noradrenaline, dopamine and 5HT, was stressed. There is a growing body of opinion that a disturbance in transmission mediated by these substances is respon-sible for endogenous depressive illness and schizophrenia, and that drugs which are effective in treating these diseases do so by correcting the disordered transmission. These views will be further developed in this chapter.

DRUGS IN PSYCHIATRY

Antidepressants

Considerable evidence has accumulated over recent years to support the monoamine hypothesis of the affective disorders. This hypothe-sis states that the level of behaviour on the depression — excitation continuum is determined by the concentration of monoamines, in certain areas of the brain which seems to be closely linked with this type of behaviour. Animal experiments in which areas of the brain are stimulated or ablated indicate that the structure most intimately concerned with emotional behaviour is the limbic system, which includes the hypothalamus, anterior thalamic nuclei, gyrus cinguli; hippocampus, amygdala and septum, and the mamillary body and fornix. These structures are rich in monoamines, and it has been reported that the concentration of 5HT is reduced in depressed patients. Experiments with drugs which modify monoaminergic transmission also support the hypothesis. Depletion of monoamine stores by reserpine leads to sedation and depression, and α-methyl p-tyrosine and α-methyldopa can have a similar effect. Reserpine depression can be antagonized by drugs which replete noradrenaline stores (e.g. levodopa) or 5HT stores (e.g. L-tryptophan) or drugs which lead to increased concentrations of free monoamines at the nerve terminal (e.g. MAOIs and tricyclic antidepressants). MAOIs in therapeutic doses have been shown to increase the concentrations of noradrenaline and 5HT in the human brain. Although there is now abundant evidence that these substances are important for the regulation of mood and motor activity, the relative contributions which each makes is still uncertain.

MAOIs

Iproniazid, the original compound in this group, was developed as an antituberculous drug, being chemically related to isoniazid. Initials trials, in 1951, revealed a central stimulant effect. A number of compounds are now in clinical use, and can be divided into *hydrazines*, including iproniazid, isocarboxazid, and phenelzine, and *non-hydrazines*, of which tranylcypromine is the only representative currently used in depression. This latter drug has in addition to its MAO inhibiting property a direct stimulant effect similar to that of amphetamine. The MAOIs which are used in treating depression inhibit both A and B variants of the enzyme. The selective MAO-B inhibitor, selegiline, is used in treating Parkinsonism (p. 87).

MAOIs are of most use when there is an endogenous component to the depression, but are also helpful in patients with a reactive or atypical depression, often with symptoms of an anxiety component. A delay of up to two weeks is usual between starting treatment with a hydrazine MAOI and the first signs of a response, and this appears to correlate with a gradually increasing concentration of brain monoamines during the first month of treatment. Tranylcypromine acts more quickly than the hydrazine derivatives. Other antidepressant drugs should be introduced with caution during the two weeks following MAOI treatment, for interactions will occur until the enzyme has been resynthesized.

The chief disadvantage of MAOI treatment is the frequency with which adverse reactions can occur, some of which are potentially lethal.

(a) Autonomic side effects, resulting from inhibition of peripheral MAO. They include dry mouth, constipation, postural hypotension, hesitancy of micturition and delayed ejaculation.

(b) Other effects, such as water retention and oedema, and increased muscle tone and reflexes.

(c) Hepatocellular damage with hydrazine drugs, producing a

mortality of up to 25% of affected patients.

(d) Hypertensive crises from interaction with other drugs and foodstuffs (see p. 39). The serious nature of these crises makes it imperative that the patient is warned of these interactions, and he should be given a card to carry with him stating the drug and its dose. Many practitioners consider that the morbidity and mortality associated with the use of MAOIs is too high to justify their routine use; indeed, in some countries they are no longer marketed.

Tricyclic and related antidepressants

These are drugs of first choice in the treatment of depression. They are most useful in endogenous depression, in which the patient's symptoms are out of all proportion to environmental stresses. They are less effective in reactive depression, and of no value when the symptoms are the result of an inadequate personality. They are often used in conjunction with electric convulsion therapy (ECT).

Table 7.1   Tricyclic and related antidepressants

Drug	Remarks
Dibenzazepine type Imipramine Desipramine Trimipramine Clomipramine Iprindole Lofepramine	Imipramine has a relatively small sedative effect and is therefore preferable for patients in whom there is no co-existent anxiety. Clomipramine, the chloro-derivative of imipramine, can be given intravenously and is said to be useful in obsessional and phobic disorders. Desipramine is the desemethylated derivative of imipramine.
Dibenzocyloheptene type Amitriptyline Nortriptyline Protriptyline Butriptyline Doxepin Dothiepin	Amitriptyline is sedative, therefore particularly useful in depressive illness accompanied by anxiety. Protriptyline acts in 5 to 10 days, the remainder in 10 to 14 days. Nortriptyline is the desemethylated derivative of amitriptyline.
Other Types Maprotiline	Maprotiline has a bridged tricyclic structure and resembles the tricyclic antidepressants in its pharmacological effects.
Mianserin	Mianserin is a tetracyclic compound which blocks presynaptic α_1 and 5HT receptors but does not inhibit monoamine reuptake.
Viloxazine	Viloxazine is a bicyclic compound with amphetamine-like central stimulant properties.
Nomifensine	An antidepressant with an activating effect, useful for the withdrawn patient.
Trazodone	Chemically unrelated to the tricyclics. Blocks 5HT receptors.

Chemically tricyclic compounds fall essentially into two types: 1. the imidobenzyl subgroup of the dibenzazepines (e.g. imipramine), and 2. the dibenzocycloheptenes (e.g. amitriptyline). Although there are no marked differences in the efficacy of the many marketed tricyclic drugs, they differ in their sedative effects, adverse effects and speed of onset of action (Table 7.1). For patients whose depressive symptoms are accompanied by anxiety, a sedative compound such as amitriptyline, nortriptyline or doxepin should be used. If taken in a single dose last thing at night they will help the patient with insomnia. Tricyclic antidepressant drugs are most likely to help those in whom physical symptoms, psychomotor slowing and disturbed thought content are prominent.

Tricyclic antidepressants block the reuptake of noradrenaline and 5HT into presynaptic nerve terminals and this has been thought to be their mode of action. However, the antidepressant effect does not appear for 10–14 days after starting treatment, whereas it is possible to demonstrate a blockade in the pressor response to tyramine (due to blockade of the uptake of tyramine, an indirectly acting sympathomimetic agent, into nerve terminals) within an hour or two of administration of the tricyclic compound. This suggests that other pharmacological actions may also contribute, and this is supported by the fact that the tetracyclic compound, mianserin, lacks uptake blocking effects; the antidepressant activity of this drug may be the result of blockade of presynaptic α_1 noradrenergic and 5HT receptors, which are inhibitory to transmitter release and whose blockade increases release. Which monoamine is more important in the antidepressant effect is uncertain. Some compounds, e.g. imipramine, selectively block noradrenaline uptake, whereas others, e.g. clomipramine, are more active on the reuptake of 5HT, but this difference does not appear to influence their clinical use. L-Tryptophan is used in conjunction with tricyclics to enhance the build-up of 5HT, but its value is controversial.

Both imipramine and amitriptyline are desmethylated to active metabolites, desipramine and nortriptyline respectively, and these may accumulate to attain plasma concentrations greater than those of the parent drugs. These compounds are extensively bound both to tissue and plasma proteins, and therefore have a large apparent volume of distribution, and are eliminated slowly from the body. It takes up to 10 days for steady state to be reached after starting treatment, and it will take a similar time for the compounds to be eliminated. Monoamine oxidase inhibitors should not, therefore, be given to a patient for two weeks after withdrawal of a tricyclic drug if the danger of an interaction is to be avoided.

Once steady has been reached, the plasma concentration of these drugs appears to be a useful guide to therapy. Carefully controlled studies have shown that an optimum antidepressant effect is seen at intermediate plasma levels, lower or higher concentrations being associated with a poorer response. At low levels, the concentration of the drug in the brain may be inadequate while at high levels it is possible that the therapeutic effect is blocked by some other pharmacological action, e.g. anticholinergic effects. It this relationship between serum level and effect is confirmed, it will become important to monitor plasma levels because failure due to over-dosing may be difficult to distinguish from that due to underdosing. Furthermore, tricyclic drugs show a wide pharmacokinetic variation between subjects. If monitoring becomes routine, it would be of advantage to prescribe desipramine or nortriptyline rather than their parent drugs because only one active substance will then need to be measured. These two compounds are entirely satisfactory for routine use. The relationship between plasma level and effect has been most thoroughly investigated for nortriptyline, the optimum therapeutic response appearing at levels of 200 to 600 nmol/1 (50 to 160 ng/ml).

The tricyclic antidepressants are useful also for the treatment of nocturnal enuresis, but are less helpful when the enuresis occurs during the day. Full antidepressant doses must be used.

Adverse effects with these drugs are frequent:

(a) Autonomic side-effects result partly from the blockade of noradrenaline uptake in sympathetic nerve terminals and partly from anticholinergic properties which these compounds possess. Tachycardia, palpitations, postural hypotension, dry mouth, hesitancy of micturition, and ocular effects, such as impaired accommodation, mydriasis and aggravation of narrow-angle glaucoma, are common.

(b) Electrocardiographic changes (flattened T waves, prolongation of the $Q - T$ interval and $S - T$ depression) and dysrhythmias have been noted both with imipramine and with amitriptyline. The latter drug has been shown to produce an increase in the incidence of sudden death in patients with pre-existing cardiac disease.

(c) Jaundice of the cholestatic type occurs rarely, particularly with iprindole.

(d) Central nervous effects include an increase in physiological tremor, drowsiness, disorientation, psychosis and hallucinations. Tricyclic drugs have a convulsant action and should be prescribed with caution in epilepsy.

(e) Dangerous interaction can occur between these drugs and the MAOIs. However, cautious combined use of the two types of compound has been advocated by some for the treatment of resistant depression.

(f) Tricyclic antidepressants potentiate the actions of directly-acting sympathomimetic amines. Dangerous hypertension can occur if local anaesthetic solutions containing a sympathomimetic vasoconstrictor substance are used in patients on tricyclics (p. 109).

The newer compounds may produce fewer adverse effects. For example, mianserin has negligible anticholinergic effects and is relatively safe for patients with heart disease. However, it has a pronounced sedative effect and causes occasional blood dyscrasias.

Amphetamines and other stimulants

Although the amphetamines release noradrenaline and dopamine from nerve terminals the central stimulant effect of these drugs is not blocked by depletion of the granular stores by reserpine, suggesting that a direct action is more important in this respect. The stimulant action effects both mental and physical performance, but the quality of these may deteriorate even though the tasks are more speedily performed. Fatigue is delayed, while sociability and confidence increase. Other central effects are isomnia, a reduction in appetite, and hyper-reflexia, while tremor results from a direct effect on skeletal muscle. Sympathetic stimulation produces tachycardia, an increased systolic blood pressure and dryness of the mouth. When given to depressed patients amphetamines produce increased alertness and elevation of mood, but the effects are often transient and may be followed by an even deeper depression. Patients in whom depression results from an inadequate personality obtain the most benefit from amphetamines, but these are the very patients who are most likely to become dependent on them. Because of the problem of abuse they should no longer be prescribed where alternative treatment exists.

Abuse, and even therapeutic use, can be followed by a withdrawal syndrome comprising fatigue, depression, hypersomnia and an increase in rapid eye movement (REM) sleep. Prolonged use can lead to the development of a chronic psychosis, resembling paranoid schizophrenia.

Other stimulant drugs include methylamphetamine, which has been given intravenously for abreaction, and methylphenidate, which has a weaker action than the amphetamines. Other related compounds, such as phenmetrazine, diethylpropion and fenfluramine are used in the treatment of obesity (Chapter 13).

Antipsychotic drugs

Whereas barbiturates have a generalized depressant effect on the central nervous system, phenothiazines and related tranquillizers exert a more selective action on certain structures which are concerned in the regulation of behaviour and wakefulness. The reticular activating system includes those parts of the midbrain reticular formation and thalamic nuclei which give rise to diffuse cortical projections concerned in maintaining a state of alertness in the cerebral cortex. Phenothiazines are selectively concentrated in these structures and block EEG arousal produced in experimental animals by sensory stimulation, possibly by an effect on the sensory collateral fibres entering the recticular formation from the lemniscal pathways. Monoamines are present in these collaterals and it may be relevant that phenothiazines block noradrenergic, dopaminergic and tryptaminergic receptors in the CNS.

Phenothiazines depress the activity of the hypothalamus and other limbic structures, most of which are particularly rich in monoamines. Their tranquillizing and antipsychotic effects, as well as their adverse effects on the extrapyramidal system correlate best with their dopamine receptor blocking properties, and therefore much attention has been devoted to the distribution of dopamine in the brain. Two pathways are particularly rich in the transmitter, the nigro-striate pathway ascending from the brain-stem to the corpus striatum (p. 82), and the mesolimbic system ascending to the nucleus acumbens and other frontal limbic structures. It seems likely that the antipsychotic effects are due to dopamine receptor blockade in the latter system whereas the extra-pyramidal effects are caused by blockade of the nigro-striate pathway. These discoveries, together with the observation that amphetamines (which stimulate central dopamine receptors) can produce a dose-related schizophreniform psychosis, have led to the hypothesis that schizophrenia may be due either to a hypersensitivity of mesolimbic dopamine receptors or to the lack of a transmitter which is normally antagonistic to dopamine. Blocking dopamine receptors would restore the correct balance and alleviate the symptoms, although a similar effect in the striatum would independently produce extra-pyramidal effects.

On the other hand, there is evidence that GABA and its synthetic enzyme, glutamic acid decarboxylase, may be deficient in the nucleus accumbens and thalamus of schizophrenic patients and it has been suggested that this deficiency may be a biochemical characteristic underlying the disorder. It is of interest in this regard that butyrophenone drugs inhibit GABA uptake into presynaptic terminals, and their potency in this correlates well with their effectiveness as antipsychotic drugs.

Phenothiazines

The first useful phenothiazine to be introduced was promethazine, which is now used only as an antihistamine and sedative drug. This was followed by chlorpromazine and subsequently a large number of related compounds. (Table 7.2). They can be classfied into three groups according the nature of a side chain on the phenothiazine nucleus:

1. aliphatic side chain (dimethylaminopropyl) derivatives
2. piperazine derivatives
3. piperidine derivatives

All these compounds have, to varying extents, blocking actions at α-adrenergic, dopaminergic, tryptaminergic and cholinergic receptors, as well as having antihistamine properties. Those derivatives with a dimethylaminopropl or piperazine side chain have marked α-adrenolytic and weak anticholinergic actions, whereas those with a piperidine side chain have the reverse. The latter derivatives produce less extrapyramidal disturbance than those of the other two groups, possibly because their greater anticholinergic effect counteracts the effect of dopamine blockade, in the same manner as atropine-like drugs have been used for treating Parkinsonism (p. 83).

The development of the phenothiazines represented the first major advance in the drug treatment of psychiatric disease, and their introduction in 1955 dramatically reversed the steady increase in the number of patients requiring admission to a longstay mental hospital. Their calming and antipsychotic properties make them particularly useful in treating schizophrenia. They can improve the blunted affect, withdrawal, thought disorder and secondary symptoms such as hallucinations and delusions, and reduce hyperactivity and aggression. It has been suggested that they 'normalize'

Table 7.2 Antipsychotic drugs

Drug	Remarks
Phenothiazines Chlorpromazine Promazine	Dimethylaminopropyl derivatives. Chlorpromazine is standard drug, but is very sedative.
Prochlorperazine Trifluoperazine Perphenazine Fluphenazine Pericyazine Thiopropazate Methotrimeprazine	Piperazine derivatives. Prochlorperazine is equivalent to chlorpromazine, but is less sedative. Useful also as an enti-emetic. Fluphenazine enanthate and decanoate are long-acting depot preparations for antipsychotic maintenance therapy. Thiopropazate is used in dyskinesias. Pericyazine has been recommended for use in character disorders.
Thioridazine	Piperidine derivative. Few extrapyramidal adverse effects.
Thioxanthenes Chlorprothixene Flupenthixol Clopenthixol	The first two are analogues of chlorpromazine and fluphenazine respectively. Flupenthixol and clopenthixol are available as decanoates for use as depot preparations.
Butyrophenones Haloperidol Trifluperidol Benperidol Droperidol	As effective as phenothiazines but extrapyramidal adverse effects frequent.
Indoles Oxypertine	Equal to phenothiazines as antipsychotic.
Diphenylbutylpiperidiness Pimozide Fluspirilene	For maintenance therapy, pimozide once daily (orally), fluspirilene once weekly (intramuscularly).

thinking. Piperazine derivatives are the most potent weight for weight, and because they have a less sedative effect they are preferable in the withdrawn patient. Chlorpromazine has the greatest sedative effect and is the drug of choice in treating violent patients. In lower dosage phenothiazines can be useful in anxiety states and psychosomatic disorders. Long-acting preparations, e.g. fluphenazine enanthate or decanoate, are valuable in reducing the relapse rate in schizophrenic patients, but their use is associated with a high incidence of adverse effects, particularly depression and extrapyramidal disturbances.

Other conditions for which phenothiazines are used include:

1. Nausea and vomiting (p. 104): chlorpromazine, prochlorperazine and trifluoperazine are the most used in this respect. Another phenothiazine, thiethylperazine, is used exclusively for this purpose. Promethazine, which possesses little antipsychotic

activity, is useful in motion sickness, probably related to its anti-cholinergic actions.

2. Allergic reactions, e.g. acute urticaria and hay fever: the powerful antihistamine effects of promethazine are most used for this purpose.

3. Pruritus: this is sometimes caused by histamine release in the skin, e.g. in acute urticaria, but in pruritus associated with jaundice it is unrelated to histamine release. Phenothiazines are antipruritic probably by a central sedative action in addition to antihistamine effects. Promethazine and trimeprazine are widely used.

4. Pain: severe pain, particularly in terminal disease, can often be controlled much better by addition of a phenothiazine.

5. Insomnia: the sedative and hypnotic effects of these compounds, particularly promethazine, can be useful.

6. Hiccough.

7 Dyskinesias: although phenothiazines can cause dyskinesias (see below) thiopropazate may be useful in controlling them (p. 88).

Adverse effects are many because phenothiazines have numerous different pharmacological actions:

(a) Peripheral autonomic effects resulting from blockade of α-adrenergic and cholinergic receptors. Postural hypotension from peripheral vasodilation is troublesome, particularly when the drug is administered parenterally. On the other hand, phenothiazines can reverse the hypotensive action of sympathetic neurone blocking drugs by preventing their uptake into the nerve terminals. Anti-cholinergic actions produce dry mouth, disturbance of accommodation, constipation and hesitancy of micturition. Quinidine-like effects on the heart are occasionally seen, producing prolongation of the $Q - T$ interval and T wave changes.

(b) Central effects resulting from modification of monoaminergic transmission. Extrapyramidal syndromes are frequently produced when high doses of phenothiazines are used for treating schizophrenia. Indeed, it is thought by some that treatment is inadequate until mild extrapyramidal disturbances are evident. Aliphatic side chain derivatives frequently produce Parkinsonism while piperazine derivatives more often cause dyskinesias. Piperidine derivatives, as mentioned above, rarely produce extra-pyramidal effects although tardive (i.e. late onset) dyskinesias can occur. The latter, which are difficult to treat, are thought to be due to a hypersensitivity of dopamine receptors consequent upon their chronic blockade. Phenothiazine-induced dyskinesias occur more often in the young, whereas Parkinsonism is the usual syndrome produced in the elderly. Because of the frequency of these side-effects, an anti-Parkinsonian drug is sometimes prescribed simultaneously when phenothiazines are required in high doses. In general, however, it is preferable to prescribe the phenothiazine alone, adding an antiParkinsonian drug if and when extrapyramidal adverse effects occur. Endocrine disturbances, such as hyperprolactinaemia, galac-torrhoea, and amenorrhoea, accompanied by a reduced urinary excretion of sex hormones and their metabolites, result probably from dopamine receptor blockade in the hypothalamus. Hypo-thermia is also due to a disturbance of hypothalamic function. Phenothiazines also have a convulsant action, the mechanism of which is unknown, and therefore they should be prescribed with caution in epilepsy.

(c) A variety of other effects, including skin rashes, pigmen-tation, photosensitivity, agranulocytosis, retinopathy and granular deposits in the lens and cornea. Cholestatic jaundice is a dose-independent hypersensitivity reaction, particularly to chlorproma-zine, and occasionally leads to permanent liver damage.

Butyrophenones

Haloperidol, trifluperidol and benperidol have proved useful in the management of psychotic patients, in particular those with a manic psychosis although they have no advantage over chlorpromazine. Weight for weight they are more potent than chlorpromazine. Another member of this group, droperidol has been used in combination with an analgesic, phenoperidine, for producing 'neuroleptanalgesia', a twilight state in which the patient can undergo a surgical procedure without pain, and subsequently have total amnesia for the event.

Because they are only weak antihistaminics, and almost completely lack anticholinergic and α-adrenolytic effects in thera-peutic doses, they infrequently produce autonomic adverse effects. Blockade of dopamine receptors frequently leads to dose-related extrapyramidal side-effects, as with phenothiazines. Depressive reactions, loss of appetite, and a syndrome including sweating, dehydration and hyperthermia can occur. Leukopenia and liver damage are occasionally seen.

Other antipsychotic drugs

The thioxanthene compounds (Table 7.2) are chemically closely related to the phenothiazines and appear to have similar pharmacological effects to their analogues. Flupenthixol appears to have a mood elevating effect, and for maintenance therapy, flupenthixol decanoate is less likely to cause depression than its fluphenazine equivalent. Oxypertine also appears equal in efficacy to phenothiazines in schizophrenia, but in lower doses it is useful in treating anxiety states. Pimozide and fluspirilene offer the advantage of once daily and once weekly administration respectively.

Anxiolytic drugs

The anxiolytic drugs differ from the phenothiazines and butyrophenones in that they have no antipsychotic activity, do not importantly affect monoamine receptors peripherally or centrally, thus producing no autonomic or extrapyramidal effects, and are more active at a spinal level, reducing transmission in polysynaptic pathways and lessening spasticity.

Benzodiazepines

The most widely used anxiolytic drugs are the benzodiazepines. Chlordiazepoxide was first marketed in the mid-1960s and rapidly became popular despite its relatively mild tranquillizing effect. It was followed soon after by diazepam, and many more have subsequently been marketed (Table 7.3). They are all 1,4-benzodiazepines except clobazam, which has 1,5-structure. Many of the 1,4-benzodiazepines are closely related metabolically. As can be seen from Figure 7.1 the major metabolite of diazepam is N-desmethyldiazepam (nordiazepam), which is pharmacologically active. The metabolites of these two compounds are temazepan and oxazepam respectively, which are marketed compounds lacking active metabolites. Potassium clorazepate is a pro-drug for N-desmethyldiazepam, and medazepam is rapidly converted to diazepam.

Because of the close interrelationships between these drugs, it can be questioned whether they differ much one from another. In terms of their effects on receptor sites, they probably do not. Current research suggests that they have a high affinity for specific 'benzodiazepine receptors' which facilitate the effects of the inhibitory transmitter GABA in the nervous system; these receptors are found in high concentration in the cerebral cortex, midbrain and limbic structures. So potent are some of the newer benzodiazepine

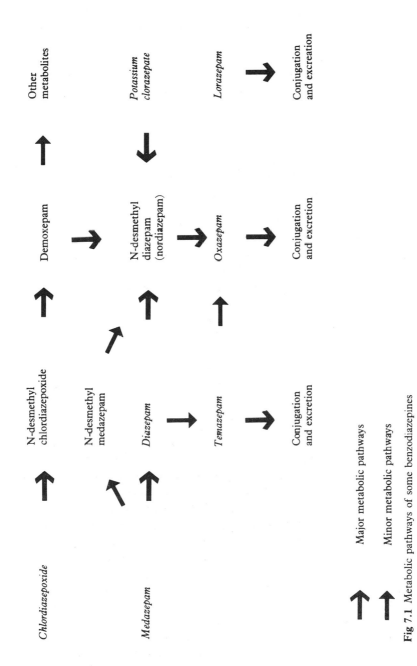

Fig 7.1 Metabolic pathways of some benzodiazepines

compounds that the presence of an endogenous ligand (with a specificity for benzodiazepine receptors resembling that of endorphins for opiate receptors) has been sought.

Table 7.3   Elimination half-lives of anxiolytic and hypnotic benzodiazepine drugs

Parent drug	Half-life	Major active metabolite(s)	Half-life
Alprazolam	Intermediate	—	—
Bromazepam	16	—	—
Chlordiazepoxide	10–20	N-desmethylchlordiazepoxide	10–20
		Demoxepam	20–70
		N-desmethyldiazepam	50–100
Clobazam	10–30	N-desmethylclobazam	30–50
Clonazepam	20–40	—	—
Clorazepate	Very short	N-desmethyldiazepam	50–100
Diazepam	20–70	N-desmethyldiazepam	50–100
Flunitrazepam*	20	—	—
Flurazepam*	Short	N-desalkylflurazepam	50–100
Ketazolam	2–3	N-desmethyldiazepam	50–100
		diazepam	32
Lorazepam	10–20	—	—
Lormetazepam	Intermediate	—	—
Medazepam	1–2	Diazepam	20–70
		N-desemthyldiazepam	50–100
Midazolam	1–3	—	—
Nitrazepam	20–40	—	—
Oxazepam	5–15	—	—
Prazepam	1.3	N-desalkylprazepam	50–100 (60)
		oxazepam	5–15
Temazepam*	5–12	—	—
Triazolam*	2–4	7 α-hydroxyderivative	

* Marketed as hypnotics (see p. 128)

In vivo, however, the effects of the various 1,4-benzodiazepines differ. Those that have the common major metabolite. N-desmethyldiazepam, namely diazepam, medazepam and clorazepate are thyldiazepam, namely diazepam, medazepam and clorazepate are indistinguishable because the metabolite is pharmacologically active and has a half-life which exceeds those of the parent compounds (Table 7.3). When diazepam is given chronically, serum levels of N-desmethyldiazepam are on average twice as high as those of diazepam itself, and therefore the pharmacokinetics of the metabolite are more important in determining the time course of the drug's effect. These are therefore long-acting preparations and are suitable as anti-anxiety drugs but not as hypnotics.

Oxazepam, temazepam and lorazepam do not have active metabolites but are conjugated and excreted. Their half-lives are shorter and they can therefore be used when a less prolonged effect is required. Temazepam is marketed as a short-acting hypnotic, for which purpose it is very suitable. Oxazepam penetrates the blood-brain barrier more slowly and is less suitable for this purpose.

Triazolam is a benzodiazepine derivative with a triazole structure. It is potent and has a half-life of only 2–4 hours. Although it has an active metabolite (Table 7.3) this also has a short half-life and therefore triazolam might be valuable as a short-acting hypnotic drug.

Clobazam is a 1,5 benzodiazepine which is claimed to possess an anti-anxiety effect without psychomotor impairment, but further assessment is needed before its place is certain.

Benzodiazepine drugs have five main uses:

1. *As anti-anxiety compounds.* There is evidence that they act selectively on the limbic system, in particular the septum, amygdala and hippocampus. In general, a longer acting drug would appear to be most suitable for this purpose, although those with a shorter half-life, e.g. oxazepam and lorazepam, have also been promoted as anti-anxiety preparations.

Benzodiazepines have become one of the most widely used groups of drugs in the Western world, and some have suggested too widely used. Although tranquillizer therapy may be fully justified when the response to life's stresses and strain is pathological, it is arguable whether normal feelings of anxiety, which may improve rather than impair performance, need treatment. Furthermore, such therapy is not without its risks. There is accumulating evidence that both psychological and physical dependence to benzodiazepine drugs can occur. The latter is due to a gradual change in the sensitivity of the bendodiazepine receptor site, leading to tolerance to the pharmacological effects of these compounds. Chronic use is associated with a gradual diminution in their hypnotic and antiepileptic effects, and the same is presumably true of their anti-anxiety action. Certainly, a clear-cut withdrawal syndrome can occur on abruptly stopping chronic benzodiazepine therapy, and includes insomnia, anxiety, tremulousness, muscle tension and twitchings, distorted perception (particularly hypersensitivity to light and sound), illusiory phenomena, and seizures. The appearance of these symptoms on stopping or reducing long-term therapy has led many patients to continue unnecessary treatment. The withdrawal syndrome is particularly severe when high doses have been given, e.g. 30 mg or more of diazepam daily; sometimes the tolerance which occurs with repeated administration leads to an escalation of dosage for exceeding the recommendations in the data sheet. Therefore, if a benzodiazepine drug is prescribed for anxiety it should be given in as low as dosage and for as short a time as possible. Furthermore, the patient should be warned against increasing the dose on his own initiative, or stopping the drug suddenly.

One advantage which benzodiazepines possess over other CNS depressant drugs is their safety in overdosage. Suicide attempts seldom succeed, even with massive doses, unless combined with another substance such as alcohol. Sedation, tiredness, muscle weakness, ataxia and diplopia are common adverse effects and, as with other tranquillizers and sedatives, driving performance is impaired and patients should be warned of this. Confusion can occur in the elderly, and this may be due to a reduced rate of metabolism, but also to an increased sensitivity of the aging brain of depressant substances.

2. *As soporific drugs* given intravenously preoperatively or during dental and endoscopic procedures. The short acting midazolam has found an important place here.

3. *As hypnotic drugs* (see p. 128).

4. *As antispasticity drugs* (p. 99) or to relieve muscle spasm associated with anxiety.

5. *As anticonvulsant drugs* given intravenously in status epilepticus (p. 95) or chronically in the management of myoclonic epilepsies (p. 94).

Other minor tranquillizers

Meprobamate has been widely used in the treatment of anxiety, particularly in the United States, where the trade name Miltown became a household word. Since the introduction of the benzodiazepines, however, its popularity has declined. Drowsiness and hypersensitivity reactions occur frequently, as do tolerance and dependence.

Several other anti-anxiety drugs are available, such as prothipendyl, benzoctamine and hydroxyzine, but they are less effective than the benzodiapines.

Lithium

Although lithium salts were used in clinical medicine many years ago, they fell into disrepute because of their toxic side-effects, but they have been reintroduced and have proved useful in the management of manic-depressive psychosis, and possibly in some patients with unipolar endogenous depression. Lithium calms manic patients and also maintains a normal mood as long as the drug is continued. Careful regulation of the dose is necessary, and frequent measurement of the plasma lithium concentration should be performed. This should be kept between 0.8 and 1.2 mmol/litre.

The drug is usually given as the carbonate or citrate. Lithium ions behave as sodium ions in excitable tissues, but cause a depression of the resting potential and spike potential. They also enhance the uptake of noradrenaline into nerve terminals and alter its metabolism in such a way as to make less of the transmitter available at the receptor. The effects of brain catecholamines are more likely to be relevant to their therapeutic effect than changes in polarization of the nerve cell.

Adverse effects are common. Tremor is almost invariable, and can be used as a clinical guide to dosage. Serum levels above 1.2 to 1.4 mmol/litre produce diarrhoea and vomiting. Tinnitus, drowsiness, ataxia, blurred vision, thirst and polyuria occur at higher levels, with confusion, nystagmus and fits when the level reaches 3 mmol/litre. Above 4 mmol/litre the outcome is usually fatal. The most serious toxic effect is on the kidney, producing a water-losing nephritis. When intoxication occurs withdrawal of lithium therapy is essential. Addition of sodium chloride to the diet has been recommended to hasten elimination of lithium, but in practice the effect is small. Goitre, sometimes accompanied by severe hypothyroidism, has been observed during lithium treatment more frequently than would be expected by chance.

Psychotomimetic drugs

These include synthetic lysergic acid derivatives, of which the diethylamide (LSD) is the most important, mescaline, which comes from the Mexican peyote cactus, and psilocybin, which is extracted from several species of mushroom. The psychic syndromes produced by these three compounds closely resemble each other. In normal man they induce:

1. Autonomic effects which are almost invariable and result from central stimulation of autonomic pathways. They include blurred vision, a rise in blood pressure, palpitations, and frequency of micturition. Other somatic symptoms occur, such as nausea, vomiting, tremulousness and ataxia.

2. Changes in mood. Anxiety and fear are common. Dramatic

swings in mood can occur, from profound depression one moment to hilarious laughter the next. Euphoria, hypomania and paranoia sometimes occur.

3. Changes in thought processes, such as difficulty in concentration, indecision, introspection and slipshod thinking.

4. Perceptual changes are not a constant feature, but are frequently seen. Vivid visual distortions or even hallucinations can occur. Auditory and tactile changes are less frequent. Distortion of body image and time sense are occasionally produced.

The pharmacological basis of these effects is uncertain. LSD is a powerful 5HT antagonist, but psilocybin is only weak in this respect, and mescaline has no anti-5HT effects at all. Furthermore, other lysergic acid derivatives are potent 5HT antagonist but have no psychotomimetic activity. It has been suggested that these drugs stimulate afferent collaterals feeding into the ascending reticular formation, which might account for changes in perception.

They have no generally accepted therapeutic uses, although they have been tried in a variety of mental diseases, and have been used for abreaction and as an adjunct to psychoanalysis. The dangers of treatment with psychotomimetic drugs, even in single doses, are substantial. Prolonged states of depression or anxiety may occur, sometimes so severe that the subject may become suicidal. Psychotic behaviour developing during the stage of acute intoxication may make the subject a danger to himself or others. Prolonged psychotic illness may ensue. The foolhardiness of experimenting with these drugs is obvious.

HYPNOTICS AND SEDATIVES

It is customary to subdivide central depressant drugs into hypnotics, sedatives and tranquillizers, partly on clinical usage of the various drugs and partly on their neuropharmacological effects in animals. Drugs which have a general depressant effect on the CNS, such as the barbiturates, have been much used in the past as hypnotics, but those which seem to be more selective in their effects on central structures, acting particularly on the ascending reticular formation and limbic system, have been promoted as tranquillizers which are claimed to reduce anxiety without producing sedation. In clinical practice, however, the relevance of this classification is less obvious, and benzodiazepine drugs are used both for hypnotic and anxiolytic purposes.

Before prescribing a hypnotic the reason for the insomnia should first be sought. If pain is the cause an analgesic should be prescribed, either alone, or in combination with a hypnotic. The latter given alone often has an 'antianalgesic' effect, making the patient with pain even more restless. The only exception to this is when the pain is accompanied by considerable anxiety. Here a sedative or tranquillizer may be helpful. In patients with respiratory failure further desensitization of the respiratory centre to an already elevated Pco_2 can precipitate CO_2 narcosis. Respiratory failure can occur in a patient in status asthmaticus, who may be critically dependent upon a raised Pco_2 to maintain respiratory drive.

Hypnotics, like tranquillizers, are amongst the most abused of drugs, both by the practitioner and by the patient. Tolerance, addiction and characteristic withdrawal symptoms have been reported with every known hypnotic, although barbiturates are probably the most potent in this respect. Withdrawal symptoms include convulsions, delirium, restlessness and insomnia accompanied by a rebound increase in REM sleep. The latter symptoms can persist for several weeks after an oversdose or on withdrawal of a regular intake of the drug, and can reinforce the patient's opinion that he cannot sleep without a nightly dose of hypnotic. Inadvertently, a sympathetic practitioner prescribing a hypnotic to tide a patient over a crisis may start a lifelong habit which is not easily broken. Hypnotics should never be prescribed without serious thought about the long-term consequences, and can usually be avoided by sensible discussion. Should one be considered necessary, a benzodiazepine compound should be chosen and it should be used for a short a time as possible or, preferably, intermittently. Barbiturates should now be considered obsolete for all but intravenous anaesthesia and epilepsy.

Benzodiazepines

Although, ideally, a hypnotic effect is an undesirable property of a tranquillizer, all the benzodiazepines have marked hypnotic actions in higher doses. The separation of benzodiazepines into hypnotics and tranquillizers (Table 7.3) is based largely on marketing convenience and pharmacokinetic properties.

In order to achieve rapid induction of sleep and a minimum of hangover effect the next day, a benzodiazepine which is quickly absorbed and which has a short elimination half-life should be selected. The drug which has been most widely used as an hypnotic is nitrazepam, but this fails to meet the ideal because it has a long half-life. Similarly, flurazepam has a long duration of action because of the slow elimination of its major metabolite, N-desalkyflurazepam. From the pharmacokinetic point of view, temazepam or, perhaps triazolam, should be selected for rapidty of action with minimum hangover. The choice, however, is determined partly by the frequency with which the hypnotic will be used. For occasional use, a drug with a long half-life may not be unacceptable, but with nightly use these compounds (or their active metabolites) may accumulate and produce continuing day-time sedation. Tolerance, however, is a factor which needs to be taken into account. With repeated administration, the hypnotic effect (and the hangover effect) diminishes until eventually only a trivial pharmacological action remains. Rebound insomnia may, of course, occur when attempts are made to stop the drug.

One major advantage of benzodiazepines is safety in overdosage. However, respiratory depression can occur, and they should therefore be avoided in patients with chronic respiratory disease. Unlike barbiturates, benzodiazepines do not induce liver enzymes, and are therefore safe in combination with oral anticoagulants.

Barbiturates

These compounds have traditionally been divided into long-, medium-, short- and ultrashort-acting drugs. The latter, by virtue of their high lipid solubility, are used as induction agents in general anaesthesia but their effect is brief because they are redistributed to other tissues, mainly fat and muscle, and they are subsequently gradually metabolized by the liver. The short- and medium-acting drugs are also degraded by the liver, and although their rates of absorption and metabolism vary slightly, this is of little practical significance. Amylobarbitone, butobarbitone, cyclobarbitone, pentobarbitone and quinalbarbitone are all similar in action as hypnotics, but their use has been largely superceded by the benzodiazepine drugs.

Barbiturates are strictly contraindicated in acute intermittent porphyria. Liver disease can impair barbiturate metabolism, although in practice the effect is not great. The powerful liver enzyme inducing property of these compounds can lead to many drug interactions, of which the most dangerous is that with oral anticoagulants. Phenobarbitone is now the only barbiturate which should be prescribed chronically (in epilepsy, p. 92).

Chloral hydrate

Although this compound was introduced just over 100 years ago it is still a useful hypnotic, especially in the young and the old. It is available only in liquid form, as the crystalline substance is hygroscopic. It is bitter to taste and irritant to the stomach. Combination of chloral hydrate with alcohol produces a potent central depressant, and this is the basis of a 'Mickey Finn'. It is largely converted by the liver to trichloroethanol, which is itself a potent hypnotic. It is one of the safest, cheapest and least toxic of hypnotics, although addiction has occasionally been reported.

Tablet forms of chloral have been introduced by esterification (Triclofos) and by combining it with phenazone (dichloralphenazone). The latter combination is reversed by liver enzymes, and the phenazone which is released can occasionally cause rashes and agranulocytosis. Phenazone, also called antipyrine, has been used as an analgesic, but is now obsolete.

Other drugs

Paraldehyde has been much used as a hypnotic, or as a sedative in disturbed patients, but its physical properties have caused it to lose favour. It is usually injected intramuscularly, but is irritant, can damage the sciatic nerve when injected badly, and cause sterile abscesses. It is exhaled in the breath, producing a penetrating and objectionable odour. It has useful anticonvulsant activity in status epilepticus (p. 96).

Glutethimide is a close relative of the barbiturates, and may be even more likely to cause a fatal outcome in overdosage. Aminoglutethimide, introduced as a hypnotic was found to cause a block in adrenal steroid synthesis, but this has been put to use therapeutically in the treatment of metastatic mammary carcinoma after the menopause or oophorectomy.

Chormethiazole, given as the base or the edisylate, is used in the elderly. Chemically related to vitamin B_1, it has a powerful, short acting hypnotic effect with minimal hangover. Its effect is variable when given orally because it undergoes extensive first pass metabolism. It is also used in acute alcohol withdrawal and, given intravenously, it has an anticonvulsant effect in status epilepticus.

Promethazine, the phenothiazine antihistamine, is a long-acting hypnotic which has been found useful in children and the elderly.

It is of value when early waking occurs. Trimeprazine is similar, and is popular as a preoperative sedative in children.

Alcohol is a useful, palatable and under-used hypnotic in the elderly.

NARCOTIC ANALGESCIS

Physiology of pain

The concept of pain as a separate modality of sensation, with its own sensory receptors, afferent fibres and ascending spinal pathways, has not been supported by recent neurophysiological research. Further theories have been based upon the electrical properties of nerve cells, and the ways in which these properties permit coding of sensory information so that common receptors and pathways may be used, but also allow decoding in higher centres. It has been recognised for some years that sensory input can be inhibited or facilitated by pathways travelling in an opposite direction to the afferent fibres, and which control transmission at the first sensory synapse. This provides a neurophysiological basis for the concept of a 'gate',which can be opened to allow information through or closed to stop it. There is some evidence that fast-conducting afferents may initiate inhibitory feedback which blocks conduction in slower afferent fibres, whereas these latter fibres can facilitate conduction. Certain pathological conditions which are characterized by pain may cause an imbalance between these two opposing forces. Non-painful sensation may become painful when the input of sensory information becomes excessive either in space or in time, or takes up a certain pattern. These changes would then cause activation of central neurones with a high threshold which are concerned with the appreciation of pain.

It is possible that centrally-acting analgesics, including opiates and some general anaesthetic agents, may act by influencing this descending (or centrifugal) control system, causing a block or change in the pattern of a potentially pain-invoking sensory input. Recent research suggests that opiate actions involve highly specific receptors in the brain, which may normally be activated by intrinsic morphine-like substances whose physiological role is that of synaptic transmission. These substances, called endorphins and enkephalins are polypeptides with amino-acid sequences corresponding with those of the C-terminal of β-lipotrophin. They are distributed widely in the CNS, but exist in particularly high concentration in the substantia gelationosa, the zone which caps the dorsal horn of the spinal cord and is probably largely involved with the modulation of sensory information. It is likely that small cells in this zone produce enkephalins which have an important role in modifying the transfer of potentially painful sensory information to ascending pathways, i.e. acting as a 'gate' (Fig. 7.2).

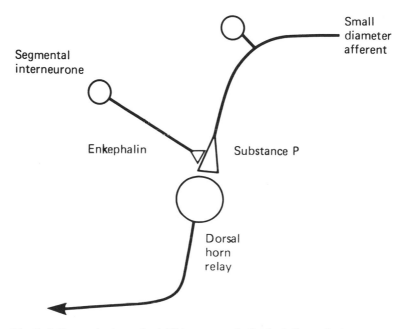

Fig. 7. 2 Proposed scheme for inhibitory control of enkephalin-producing interneurones in the substantia gelationosa over primary afferent fibres producing the excitatory transmitter, substance P.

β-Endorphin and methionine enkephalin can produce profound analgesia when injected intraventricularly in animals and intrathecally in man. The specific opiate antagonist, naloxone, can lower pain threshold in some people, can increase post-operative dental pain, and reverse the analgesic effect produced by a placebo and by acupuncture. These observations suggest that endorphins and enkephalins may play an important physiological role in pain control, and that narcotic analgesics act by mimicking these endogenous substances. They act on opioid receptors in the CNS; these receptors are subclassified into mu receptors mediating analgesia, delta receptors causing respiratory depression, kappa receptors responsible for sedation, and sigma receptors producing dysphoria and hallucinations. Some of the newer opioid drugs are thought to be more selective on mu receptors than the traditional compounds.

From the practical point of view there are two types of pain, visceral and somatic. The former is a dull, poorly localized pain, and is not helped by non-narcotic drugs, whereas the latter is sharply defined, is usually relieved by a mild analgesic and seldom requires an opiate. This, perhaps, is fortunate as there are many chronic musculoskeletal conditions which require analgesic treatment over many years. The use of opiate drugs should not be contemplated unless the painful condition is of very limited duration. e.g. postoperative, or accompanies terminal disease such as cancer, when addicition is of no concern.

Pain is a symptom of underlying pathology and is of vital diagnostic importance. Its uncritical relief is to be deplored, as a valuable sign of worsening disease will be lost. Treatment should be given only when a firm diagnosis has been made and an alternative means of assessment is available.

As in many other areas of therapeutics a placebo effect is important in the treatment of pain. One study showed that capsules containing 10 mg of morphine were only slightly superior to placebo in relieving postoperative pain, and the placebo itself gave relief in almost one third of the patients. In another study of experimental pain in fit adults, 50 mg of pethidine intramuscularly was indistinguishable from saline, and 100 mg was only slightly superior.

Pharmacology of narcotic (opioid) analgesics

These compounds have effects on many different tissues, probably resulting from influencing important, but poorly understood, intracellular enzyme system. In brief, the following pharmacological actions are seen:

(a) Central effects, including analgesia, euphoria and drowsiness. An elevation of the pain threshold seems to occur, but, in addition, the patient's attitude and emotional response to the pain is altered. This euphoriant effect is the reason why opiates are drugs of abuse.

(b) Respiratory depression is produced by an effect on the respiratory centre, lowering its sensitivity to changes in $P\text{CO}_2$.

(c) Depression of the cough reflex. Opiates are included in a number of cough mixtures.

(d) Nausea and vomiting particularly with morphine, resulting from stimulation of the chemoreceptor trigger zone. This occurs every time in some patients, but never in others. Larger doses of morphine inhibit vomiting by an action on the emetic centre.

(e) Miosis, from stimulation of the parasympathetic outflow responsible for pupillo-constriction. Pethidine and its analogues lack this effect.

(f) Increase in smooth muscle tone and a reduction in its motility, causing constipation, spasm of the sphincter of Oddi and bronchoconstriction.

(g) Hypotension, from depression of ganglionic transmission, producing vasodilatation.

(h) Histamine release occurs occasionally, especially with morphine, causing urticaria and pruritus.

Individual compounds. A wide variety of compounds are available, some being naturally-occurring alkaloids and others semisynthetic or synthetic. Discussion will be confined to the more important representatives. Essentially they can be divided into four groups:

1. Morphine group, including morphine itself, the semisynthetic opiate diamorphine (heroin), and the synthetic opioid compounds, levorphanol, dextromoramide, phenazocine and pentazocine, which closely resemble morphine in strcture and actions. Morphine is still the most used of these drugs but it frequently produces nausea and vomiting. Diamorphine is preferred by some on the grounds that it less often causes these effects, and also rarely constipates. It has less tendency to produce hypotension and for this reason is often chosen in patients who have had a myocardial infarction, for the mortality in this condition is directly related to the occurrence of hypotension. It also produces more euphoria, and this may be the reason why it appears to be more addicting than morphine. In the U.S.A. and many other countries its use for medical purposes is illegal, although this seems to have contributed little to solving the problem of addiction.

Levorphanol and dextromoramide are well absorbed by mouth, and are valuable in the management of chronic pain in terminal disease. Levorphanol is the longer-acting of the two.

Phenazocine is more potent than morphine, but in equianalgesic doses it possibly produces less sedation, vomiting and hypotension than morphine. Its respiratory depressant effect is greater, and it is not the drug of choice in obstetrics or in patients with chest disease. Unlike morphine, it does not affect the sphincter of Oddi.

Pentazocine seems to have a low addiction potential, and for this reason is not controlled by the Misuse of Drugs Act. A withdrawal syndrome occurs, but is mild compared with morphine withdrawal. Pentazocine was developed originally as a narcotic antagonist and like them it can cause hallucinations, bad dreams and thought disturbances, but not as often. Nevertheless the frequency with which they occur is a major disadvantage, and may, in part, account for the low addiction potential of the drug. It is not the drug of choice in myocardial infarction, for it increase pulmonary and systemic blood pressure and left ventricular work. It has a potency somewhere between codeine and morphine. It has an unpredictable effect orally and is usually given parenterally.

Papaveretum is a mixture of purified opium alkaloids in proportions which occur naturally. Almost 50% is morphine, so 20 mg of papaveretum is approximately equivalent to 10 mg of morphine in terms of its analgesic effects. It has no particular advantages.

2. Pethidine group, including pethidine and phenoperidine, but the latter drug has been used mainly for neuroleptanalgesia. They are synthetic, and although their structures bear only slight resemblance to that of morphine they have many actions in common with this drug. Pethidine is less potent than morphine, but in equianalgesic doses it produces less constipation, nausea and vomiting. Although it was initially developed as a spasmolytic drug, and it has been claimed to have atropine-like effects when used as an analgesic, these properties are weak or non-existent, and it is not superior to morphine for pain of visceral origin. It does not affect the pupil, and does not reduce cough. It has a shorter duration of action than morphine and may be disappointing orally. It produces less sedation and euphoria, but addiction occurs readily.

Phenoperidine is more potent than morphine in its analgesic and respiratory depressant effects. It produces little sedation, but when given with the butyrophenone, droperidol, it produces the twilight state of neuroleptanalgesia.

3. Methadone group, including methadone and dipipanone. These are synthetic heptanones, only remotely related chemically to morphine. They produce much less sedation, euphoria, respiratory depression and miosis. Methadone is useful for controlling morphine withdrawal symptoms in addicts undergoing treatment. Both drugs are satisfactorily absorbed orally, and are used in the management of chronic pain in terminal disease. Dextropropoxyphene is a mild analgesic related structurally to methadone, and is popular for treating mild pain. Alone, its effect are significantly inferior to those of aspirin, but in combination with aspirin or

paracetamol (Distalgesic contains the latter) it is a useful analgesic. There is concern over its ability to produce addiction, and over-dosage can be difficult to manage because the patient's state may fluctuate widely, showing features of stimulation and depression in which respiratory depression can be predominant. Furthermore, interaction with alcohol can be hazardous.

4. Codeine group, including the naturally occurring alkaloid codeine, the semisynthetic dihydrocodeine and pholcodine. Codeine is a weak analgesic to which dependence rarely occurs. It is used in somatic pain, as a cough suppressant and as an antidiarrhoeal (as codeine phosphate). A variety of commercial preparations contain a low dose of codeine in combination with aspirin or paracetamol. Full analgesic doses of codeine produce too much constipation for long term treatment to be practical. Dihydro-codeine has an analgesic potency somewhere between codeine and morphine. Orally it is often more effective than pethidine, but like codeine it constipates and can produce unpleasant dizziness. Phol-codine is used only as an antitussive.

Narcotic antagonists

Nalorphine, levallorphan and naloxone are structurally related to morphine but have only weak analgesic properties. They can coun-teract the respiratory depressant effects of most narcotic drugs, and are invaluable as specific antagonists in narcotic overdosage. Nal-oxone is the drug of choice because it lacks respiratory depressant properties, whereas nalorphine and levallorphan will produce severe depression if given inadvertently to a patient who has over-dosed with hypnotic drugs rather than opiates. Nalorphine, but not levallorphan, can induce a severe withdrawal syndrome in a narcotic addict. In a belief that levallorphan antagonizes the respiratory depressant but not the analgesic effect of pethidine, these two compounds have been combined as 'Pethilorfan' for obstetric anal-gesia in an attempt to prevent depression of breathing in the newborn while providing good analgesia in the mother. In practice, this preparation seems no better in this respect than pethidine alone.

Narcotic antagonists have analgesic effects of their own, but they can cause hallucinations and unpleasant affective and thought disturbances if given in sufficient dosage to produce useful analgesia.

Mixed agonist/antagonist drugs

Some of the newer compounds have mixed agonist/antagonist activity which gives them a more selective action on the receptors mediating analgesia. They have less respiratory depressant activity and are less liable to cause addiction.

Buprenorphine is used as a long-acting analgesic in place of morphine. It has minimal effects on the cardiovascular system, a relatively low addiction potential, and is incompletely reversed by naloxone. Butorphanol is similar. Meptazinol is a drug with a lower potency but it can be given orally or moderate pain.

Other drugs

Nefopam is an analgesic unrelated to the narcotic analgesics, with an unknown mode of action. It may be useful for persistent pain, but hepatotoxicity occurs.

Treatment of acute pain

Parenteral preparations are required for treating acute pain. If they are injected subcutaneously or intramuscularly into a shocked patient, they are poorly absorbed from vasoconstricted tissues. Under these circumstances they should be injected slowly intravenously until effective analgesia has been achieved. This method is also useful for determining the dose of drug required to produce pain relief with subsequent intramuscular maintenance therapy.

The choice of drug depends largely upon the severity of the pain. Morphine and heroin are the most effective in severe pain, but phenazocine is a useful alternative. Their various advantages and disadvantages have been considered above. Pethidine and pentazocine are unable to produce analgesia equivalent to that of morphine, however large the dose, and are therefore suitable only for milder pain. Pethidine has been the most popular analgesic in obstetrics for a number of years because it depresses the respiratory centre of the newborn less than morphine and is shorter in its duration of action. Recent trials have suggested that pentazocine may be as satisfactory as pethidine for this purpose. Dihydrocodeine is satisfactory in mild pain, but it constipates on repeated dosage.

Acute pain is often accompanied by anxiety, which can in turn make the pain worse. Morphine and heroin are particularly useful in this circumstances, for they produce marked sedation and euphoria which contribute substantially to the resulting analgesia. It is unnecessary to administer a tranquillizer or sedative at the same time. Indeed, it is a hazardous practice to inject an opiate and another central depressant drug simultaneously, for the respiratory depressant effect of the opiate may be potentiated to an extent where repiratory arrest occurs.

Powerful narcotic drugs should be prescribed for only a few days for postoperative pain and other acutely painful conditions, because dependence becomes a risk if treatment is continued longer. A withdrawal syndrome is usually seen when morphine is stopped after about 1 to 2 weeks of continuous use.

Treatment of chronic pain

In the management of pain accompanying terminal disease, oral treatment is desirable where possible. An aqueous solution of morphine or diamorphine given orally is satisfactory as a first choice of narcotic analgesic. The object of treatment should be to prevent pain rather than to suppress it each time it returns. The narcotic should be given four-hourly in a dose which has been titrated to free the patient of pain. Tolerance and addiction are seldom a problem. Drowsiness usually passes within a few days, and respiratory depression is rarely troublesome. Constipation is frequent and may require a regular laxative.

As alternatives to morphine, drugs of moderate strength such as papaveretum or dipipanone can be used. A stronger narcotic may become necessary, when levorphanol, dextromoramide or phenazocine are suitable. Methadone is cumulative and difficult to manage, and pethidine and pentazocine have too short a duration of action and are poorly effective.

Parenteral analgesics may be necessary when intractable nausea and vomiting do not respond to anti-emetics. Diamorphine is best because it is more soluble than morphine and a smaller volume can be injected.

Phenothiazines have been used to potentiate the analgesic action of opiates, although the effectiveness of this remains to be proven. However, phenothiazines will control nausea and vomiting produced either by the disease or by the opiate. Mixtures of cocaine, heroin and alcohol have been used for many years, but there is no evidence that cocaine reduces drowsiness or enhances mood, and some patients dislike the alcohol.

Non-analgesic uses

Because of their ability to produce sedation and euphoria, opiates have long been used for premedication. Other marginal benefits result from their use in this situation, including a lessening of mucus and saliva production, and a reduced incidence of cardiac and respiratory irregularities. Respiratory depression, nausea, vomiting and constipation are drawbacks, however, and benzodiazepine drugs are used increasingly for premedication.

Similarly, morphine has been used widely for sedating patients with haematemesis, but as these patients are often hypovolaemic and shocked intramuscular injections can be poorly absorbed.

The dyspnoea produced by pulmonary oedema (e.g. paroxysmal nocturnal dyspnoea) is greatly reduced by morphine, and improved ventilation assists reabsorption of the fluid from the alveoli. But it is critical to distinguish between the dyspnoea of pulmonary oedema and that of status asthmaticus, for morphine may precipitate respiratory failure in the latter condition. Fortunately, the development of potent diuretic drugs such as frusemide, bumetanide and ethacrynic acid have made the administration of morphine unnecessary in pulmonary oedema, and therefore the danger resulting from misdiagnosis is eliminated.

Contraindications

Narcotic analgesics should never be used in the following conditions:

(a) Respiratory disease. Respiratory failure can result.

(b) Liver disease. Hepatic encephalopathy may ensue.

(c) Hypothyroidism, hypopituitarism or Addison's disease. Coma may be precipitated.

(d) Raised intracranial tension. Coma may be precipitated.

(e) Head injury. Valuable pupil signs may be lost.

Patients receiving a MAOI should not be given a narcotic analgesic, for the effects of the analgesic can be greatly exaggerated, producing excitation, rigidity, coma, hyperpyrexia and changes in blood pressure, more commonly hypotension.

Narcotic dependence

Dependence can be induced in any subject given a narcotic in sufficient dosage for a sufficient time, but addiction, with all its physical, psychological and social implication, occurs only in those who need an escape from reality. A discussion of these problems is beyond the scope of this book.

Withdrawal of morphine from an addict produces a withdrawal syndrome, comprising restlessness, anxiety, yawning, sweating and lacrimation. After about 24 hours cramps, muscle twitching, vomiting and diarrhoea begin, and reach a peak at 48 to 72 hours. Insomnia and hallucinations occur. The syndrome settles after 5 to 10 days. Injection of an opiate antagonist can precipitate this syndrome in an addict, and it has been used as a diagnostic test, but it is dangerous unless performed by one experienced in this field. Cross-dependence between many different opiates occurs, and this is utilized in controlling morphine or heroin withdrawal symptoms with methadone.

FURTHER READING

Kruk Z L, Pycock C J 1979 Neurotransmitters and drugs. Croom Helm, London
Lader M 1980 Introduction to psychopharmacology. A Scope Publication, Upjohn, Kalamazoo

8

Drugs on the heart

DRUGS WITH POSITIVE INOTROPIC ACTIVITY

Digitalis and related glycosides

These agents are widely distributed in nature. Chemically they are made up of an aglycone ring structure which determines the drug's pharmacological activity and one to and four sugar molecules which influence water solubility, cell penetration and pharmacokinetic properties. The glycosides most commonly used in clinical practice are digoxin, digitoxin, and ouabain.

Mechanism of action. Digitalis glycosides are thought to inhibit the sodium pump in the sarcolemma by acting on the enzyme sodium-potassium ATPase. This allows the intracellular sodium concentration to rise, thus increasing the free calcium ion concentration and the contractile force achieved at any given left ventricular filling pressure.

Conduction in the bundle of His is depressed by digitalis glycosides, with a subsequent increase in atroventricular conduction time and a lengthening of the PR interval on the electrocardiogram. Other effects on the electrocardiogram are depression of the horizontal ST segment, followed by a biphasic T wave. Ultimately the T wave becomes entirely inverted leading steeply from the depressed ST segment. The QT interval is shortened due to a reduction in the duration of ventricular systole.

Digitalis increases vagal tone in the heart resulting in slowing of the sinoatrial node rate and further depression of conduction in the bundle of His.

Pharmacokinetics. Digoxin is incompletely absorbed after oral administration and although there is no first-pass effect, bioavailability is between 65 and 75%. The degree of plasma protein binding is low and the drug is distributed widely throughout the body with much higher myocardial concentrations than plasma concen-

142

trations. On average, 70% of the drug is excreted unchanged in the urine with an elimination half-life of around 42 hours. Clearance of digoxin decreases in hypothyroidism, congestive cardiac failure and chronic renal failure. It also declines in the elderly due to the decline in renal function.

Ouabain is very poorly absorbed after oral administration and is normally given by slow intravenous injection. It is predominantly excreted unchanged in the urine with a half-life of approximately 20 hours. Digitoxin is almost completely absorbed after oral administration. It is about 90% bound in plasma, although this can be reduced in renal disease. 70% of the drug is metabolized and the remainder excreted unchanged in the urine. The half-life of elimination is around about 7 days and the drug undergoes extensive enteropatic recirculation. The half-life is unaffected by renal impairment.

Adverse effects. Most of the adverse effects of digitalis glycosides are dose-dependent and may be seen in up to a quarter of patients taking the drug. The commonest symptoms are those affecting the gastrointestinal tract such as anorexia, nausea, vomiting and a change in bowel habit, usually diarrhoea. Neurological symptoms are also common and include headache, fatigue, insomnia, confusion, depression and vertigo. Abnormalities of colour vision and amblyopia and photophobia are sometimes seen.

Digitalis overdosage may lead to almost any cardiac arrhythmia particularly ventricular ectopic beats. These may progress to coupling with an ectopic beat following closely on a normally generated contraction. Bradycardia supraventricular and ventricular arrhythmias may be seen and AV nodal conduction impairment can lead to heart block. At any particular plasma digoxin concentration, toxicity is commoner in patients who are hypokalaemic, hypomagnesaemic or hypercalcaemic. Hypothyroid patients are also more sensitive, while hyperthyroid patients appear to be relatively resistant to the effects of cardiac glycosides. The elderly and those who are hypoxic are also at greater risk. In the absence of these complicating factors, optimal drug effect usually occurs above plasma concentration of 1.3 nanomoles per litre. Toxicity occurs relatively frequently above a plasma concentration of 2.6 nanomoles per litre. Quinidine, spironolactone, amiodarone and verapamil may reduce renal digoxin clearance by competing with an active tubular secretary mechanism for digoxin in the distal convoluted tubule. Toxicity may therefore result at lower daily digoxin dosage when these drugs are prescribed concurrently. Hypokalaemia induced by other agents (e.g. diuretics) may also enhance the effect of cardiac glycosides.

Therapeutic indications. The major clinical use for digitalis glycosides is in atrial fibrillation when it slows the ventricular rate and occasionally allows reversion to sinus rhythm. It may be of benefit in other supraventricular tachycardias, but is best avoided in patients with Wolff-Parkinson-White syndrome. It may have temporary benefit in patients with heart failure not associated with atrial fibrillation, but this benefit may not be sustained subsequently. It should be used with great caution in patients with heart block, since this may be worsened. In hypertropic obstructive cardiomyopathy, the positive inotropic effect can result in a increase in the obstruction to outflow. Digoxin appears to be of little value in heart failure due to cor pulmonale or acute cardiomyopathies.

Ouabain is sometimes used in emergency since it may exert a beneficial action within half an hour, whereas the effect of digoxin may take up to 1 to 5 hours. Some physicians prefer digitoxin because of its longer duration of action, but is more difficult to adjust the dose because the clearance of the compound is difficult to predict in any particular individual. Since digoxin clearance appears to be relatively closely related to renal function, it is easier to tailor the dose to the patient's needs and digoxin should be considered for routine use. If rapid effect is required, a loading dose is necessary because of the long half-life of digoxin. When very rapid control is needed then digoxin can be given intravenously, but it must be given slowly. An oral loading dose can be used in less urgent situations but in many cases the patient can be started directly on a maintenance dose.

Glucagon

Glucagon is a polypeptide hormone produced by the α-cells of the pancreatic islets. It has marked hyperglycaemic properties and in addition has been shown to release insulin, growth hormone, thyroid hormones, calcitonin, parathormone and catecholamines from their respective endocrine glands. It increases the force of cardiac contraction by increasing myocardial adenyl cyclase activity without stimulating the β-adrenoceptor, and therefore its action is not blocked by β-receptor antagonists. It also increases heart rate, but its maximal inotropic action is relatively weak. Although nausea and vomiting occur relatively frequently with its use in a dose-related fashion, they may be partly controlled by phenothiazine pretreatment. It rarely induces arrhythmias and is potentially useful in patients who are shocked because of β-receptor antagonist overdose, until the appropriate dose of β-receptor agonist has been found by dose-titration.

β-adrenoceptor agonists

Normal myocardial contractility and function are dependent on sympathetic drive. In congestive cardiac failure the myocardium becomes depleted of noradrenaline and reflex sympathetic activity can no longer produce the increased performance required to compensate for the myocardial failure. However, if catecholamines with predominant β-receptor stimulating activity are given, sympathetic drive may be increased and function improved.

Isoprenaline is a non-selective stimulant of β_1 and β_2 receptors and has no α-receptor agonist activity. It is poorly bioavailable after oral administration because of extensive metabolism in the liver and gut, but after intravenous infusion, it increases cardiac output nad heart rate, which is further increased by reflex action by the fall in peripheral resistance produced by the β_2 mediated relaxation of vascular smooth muscle. It has been used in the treatment of bradycardia due to heart block either acutely or for long term treatment to prevent Stokes-Adams attacks. In both circumstances, however, insertion of a pacemaker is preferable. Its use in the treatment of heart failure has largely been superceded by the use of dopamine and dobutamine since they have less tendency to provoke arrhythmias, particularly ventricular arrhythmias at therapeutic doses.

Dopamine is a naturally occurring precursor of noradrenaline which at pharmacological doses stimulates dopamine receptors and β_1 receptors and then at higher doses α_1 receptors. Stimulation of dopamine receptors leads to a selective increase of blood flow in the renal, mesenteric cerebral and coronary beds. β_1 stimulation produces an inotropic effect. At higher doses the α-agonist reaction leads to peripheral vasoconstriction and fall in renal blood flow. Although it is less likely to cause arrhythmias than isoprenaline, they are still possible and it should not be used in patients with phaeochromocytoma or in patients in whom the myocardium has been sensitized to catecholamines by cyclopropane or one of the halogenated anaesthetics (e.g. halothane). It is rapidly metabolized after oral administration and must be given intravenously by infusion because of its short half-life of elimination. It is partly metabolized by monoamine oxidase and the dose should be reduced in patients on monoamine oxidase inhibitors.

Dobutamine is a synthetic product with predominant β_1 agonist activity. It is therefore a positive inotrope which produces little rise in heart rate. It does not stimulate dopamine receptors and has only minor action on α-receptors. It is not active orally and must be given by continuous intravenous infusion because of its short half-life of elimination. Ventricular arrhythmias may occur less frequently with dobutamine than with dopamine and dobutamine appears to be more effective in reducing left ventricular filling pressure. Dobutamine and dopamine have been combined in cardiogenic shock to obtain the pharmacological benefits of both drugs and improved clinical response.

Prenalterol is a relatively selective β_1 agonist which improves myocardial contractility but must be given intravenously, so like the other sympathomimetic agents it is only useful for short-term treatment.

ANTIARRHYTHMIC DRUGS

Drugs which supress arrhythmias have been divided into four classes depending on their predominant mode of action.
1. Membrane stabilizing drugs
2. β-receptor blocking drugs
3. Drugs affecting the action potential duration
4. Calcium antagonists

Class 1 antiarrhythmic agents

These drugs share the common property of raising the threshold of the myocardium to stimulation by a direct membrane stabilizing action. Drugs within this class are further subdivided into Class 1A agents and Class 1B agents. Class 1A agents slow down phase 0 of the action potential in spontaneously depolarizing cells by slowing sodium influx and thereby increasing the action potential duration (Fig. 8.1).

Class 1B agents shorten phase 3 by enhancing the rate of potassium efflux and therefore decrease the action potential duration. However, both groups of agents increase the effective refractory period relative to the action potential duration so that conducting tissue is resistant to depolarization for a relatively longer period. Both agents also reduce the automaticity of spontaneously depolar-

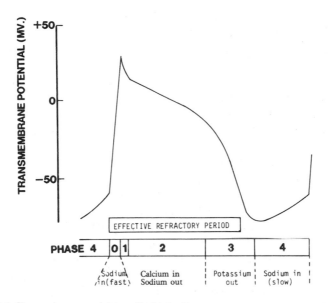

Fig. 8.1 Fast action potential in a Purkinje fibre.

izing cells in the heart by slowing the rate of depolarization during phase 4, although class 1A agents also raise the threshold for depolarization and so have a greater effect.

Class 1A agents

Quinidine. Quinidine is a stereo-isomer of quinidine which slows the rate of sodium entry across the cell membrane on depolarization. Action potential duration is increased and conduction depressed with a 50% prolongation of the QRS width and increased P–R and Q–T intervals. Myocardial contractility may also be impaired but resting heart rate may increased slightly due to its anticholinergic effects.

Quinidine is relatively well absorbed from the gastro-intestinal tract and 80% is metabolized in the liver, the rest being excreted in the urine. Clearance is reduced in patients with cirrhosis, congestive cardiac failure and in the elderly. Two thirds of patients receiving the drug develop toxicity particularly nausea, vomiting and diarrhoea and other dose-dependent effects include vertigo, tinnitus, deafness, blurred vision and mental confusion. Disorders of cardiac rhythm such as atrioventricular block, ventricular ectopics and ventricular fibrillation may also occur. The drug should not be used if the QT interval is already increased and should be stopped if the QRS interval increases to 0.12 seconds or more.

Dose-independent toxicity includes urticaria and anaphylaxis and thrombocytopenic purpura. A 200 mg test dose is therefore given and the patient carefully observed for evidence of hypersensitivity before oral therapy is started. Because of its toxicity the drug is now used less frequently than it was.

Disopyramide. Disopyramide has similar electrophysiological effects to quinidine, although its effects on QRS duration and QT interval are less pronounced. It has a significant negative inotropic effect and marked anticholinergic properties. After oral administration it is well absorbed and half of the drug is cleared by hepatic metabolism, the remainder being excreted in the urine. Reduced clearance is therefore associated with renal as well as liver disease. The anticholinergic effects of disopyramide may cause urinary retention or acute glaucoma, particularly in the elderly. Gastrointestinal problems are less common than with quinidine and cardiac toxicity is not common in patients with relatively normal hearts. Patients with sick sinus syndrome do not tolerate the drug well, and it should be used with caution in patients with cardiomegaly because of the risks of precipitation of heart failure. Disopyramide is predominantly used for treatment of ventricular arrhythmias but is less effective against atrial arrhythmias except those associated with Wolff-Parkinson-White syndrome.

Procainamide. Procainamide has similar electrophysical actions to quinidine but has less anti-cholinergic activity than procainamide or disopyramide. It is well absorbed from the gastrointestinal tract. Just over half of the drug is cleared by renal elimination and the rest is metabolized by N-acetylation to N-acetyl procainamide which itself has anti-arrhythmic activity. Clearance of the drug is therefore lower in slow acetylators and those with renal dysfunction. The drug can cause gastrointestinal symptoms and very rarely, agranulocytosis after prolonged treatment. An important problem is the onset of a lupus erythematosus-like syndrome which appears to occur earlier and with lower total cumulative doses in slow acetylators. Because of the drug's short half-life it must be given either frequently or in the form of a slow release preparation. Procainamide, like the other Class 1A agents, may cause a polymorphic ventricular tachycardia termed *'torsades de pointes'*. This arrhythmia may be associated with the effect of Class 1A drugs on the QT interval and is commoner with quinidine than with the other two agents. The potential therapeutic role of the metabolite N-acetyl procainamide is still being studied. It has a longer half-life than procainamide, is excreted predominantly unchanged in the urine and does not appear to be associated with drug induced lupus erythematosus.

Class 1B agents

Class 1B agents shorten action potential duration and do not affect the QRS complex or QT interval. They are more effective in ventricular than supraventricular arrhythmias.

Lignocaine. Lignocaine is the most widely used agent for the acute treatment of ventricular arrhythmias. Although well absorbed, its bioavailability is variable and poor because of large presystemic elimination. It is therefore given intramuscularly, or more commonly by intravenous infusion. It is 70% bound in plasma particularly to α-1-acid glycoprotein (AAG) so that plasma protein binding can be increased in patients with high AAG concentrations due to inflammatory disease, recent myocardial infarction or chronic renal failure. The drug is virtually completely cleared by hepatic metabolism in a non-restrictive fashion and clearance falls in hepatic cirrhosis and in congestive cardiac failure because of reduced liver blood flow. The half-life is approximately 2 hours in the normal individual, but is increased in heart failure, chronic liver disease and after prolonged administration of the drug. The clearance of lignocaine appears to fall progressively after myocardial infarction but at least part of this is due to an increase in AAG so that the increase in total blood levels after constant intravenous infusion does not reflect the change in free drug concentration which increases much more modestly. Because the drug is extensively and rapidly distributed within tissues a loading dose in necessary to prevent early sub-therapeutic plasma drug levels. One approach is to give a 75 mg loading dose over 2 minutes, followed by an infusion of 8 mg per minute for 20 minutes. The patient can then be started on a maintenance dose of 2 mg per minute, although this dose must be reduced in patients with congestive cardiac heart failure and liver disease. The adverse effects are predominantly dose-dependent and affect the CNS. Disorientation, parathaesiae and drowsiness may be followed by coma and convulsions. Effects on the cardiovascular system are rare but include sinus arrest, asystole and atrioventricular block. The drug should therefore be used with care in patients with pre-existing conduction disturbances. Lignocaine has very little negative inotropic effect at therapeutic plasma concentrations and dose-independent hypersensitivity reactions are extremely rare.

Mexiletine. Mexiletine is similar to lignocaine but has a high oral bioavailability and can be administered orally as well as intravenously. It is highly protein bound and is almost completely cleared by liver metabolism so that toxicity is more likely in patients with liver dysfunction. Unlike lignocaine, however, it undergoes a restrictive elimination and clearance is much less dependent on liver blood flow than on hepatic enzyme activity. The half-life of elimination is approximately 12 hours and the drug is usually given 3 or 4 times daily.

Adverse effects of mexiletine are relatively common and dose-dependent. They include gastrointestinal intolerance and CNS symptoms similar to those caused by lignocaine. The therapeutic index is small so that the drug dosage much be carefully titrated to prevent toxicity but, like lignocaine, mexiletine only rarely causes cardiac toxicity.

Tocainide. Tocainide is structurally very similar to lignocaine but undergoes little presystemic metabolism and therefore can be given orally. It is poorly protein bound and is cleared by hepatic metabolism (60%) and renal elimination. The half-life is 12 to 15 hours so that the drug can be given in 2 or 3 divided doses. It causes a similar spectrum of adverse effects to lignocaine and mexiletine and dose independent toxicity, although described, is rare. It may be better tolerated than mexiletine but may also be less effective.

Phenytoin. Phenytoin has antiarrhythmic as well as anticonvulsant activity. It shortens the action potential duration and is particularly effective in suppressing digitalis induced ventricular arrhythmias. Its adverse effects after prolonged oral use are dealt with elsewhere, but for antiarrhythmic purposes it is normally given by intravenous infusion. Adverse effects by this route of administration include bradycardia, hypotension, AV block and asystole which are less likely when the drug is given slowly.

Class 2 antiarrhythmic agents

β-blockers exert their antiarrhythmic effects through their ability to block the arrhythmogenic effects of circulating catecholamines and it is by this mechanism that they slow sinus rate and prolong atrioventricular conduction. It is unlikely that the membrane stabilizing activity is therapeutically important at conventional doses of those β-blockers which possess this activity in vitro (e.g. propranolol).

β-Blockers are effective in preventing sinus tachycardia and are used in patients in whom the tachycardia is distressing (e.g. in hyperthyroidism). In incipient heart failure, sinus tachycardia is a compensatory mechanism produced by catecholamine drive and β-blockade may lead to serious heart failure, even after only one or two doses of the drug. β-blockers have also been used in the treatment and prophylaxis of paroxsysmal supraventricular tachycardia. Although digitalis is still the drug of choice in controlling ventricular rate in atrial fibrillation, propranolol may be given after the patient is digitalised if digoxin toxicity prevents the dose of digoxin from being increased to satisfactorily control ventricular rate, particularly after exercise. Ventricular arrhythmias in phaeochromocytoma and during anaesthaesia respond well to β-blockers, and they are sometimes effective against exercise related ventricular tachycardia. They are less effective against other chronic ventricular arrhythmias. Their benefit in reducing mortality after myocardial infarction may be related to the ability to suppress serious ventricular arrhythmias. Apart from the effect on contractile activity which has been mentioned previously, β-blockers may precipitate conduction disturbances, particularly in those patients with pre-existing sino-atrial or AV conduction disturbance, and they should not be used in patients with second or third degree heart block.

Class 3 antiarrythmic agents

These agents prolong action potential duration in atrial and ventricular conducting tissue by slowing phase 3 of the action potential. Although one of the β-blocking agents, sotalol, has Class 3 activity, the most commonly used agent is amiodarone.

Amiodarone. Amiodarone prolongs the refractory period of the atria, ventricles and AV node and any accessory AV pathways, and slows sinus rate. It may also act indirectly by non-competitively blocking sympathetic stimulation. The drug can be given by oral administration but bioavailability is low because of poor absorption. It is widely distributed throughout tissues and has a slow elimination half-life of over 30 days. Clearance is by hepatic metabolism. Adverse effects appear to be dose-related and include hyper-or hypothyroidism, corneal micro deposits, a bluish discolouration of the skin and cutaneous photosensitivity. Nausea and vomiting may be troublesome. Peripheral neuropathy has also been recorded but the most life threatening complication is pulmonary infiltration which may lead to respiratory failure.

Amiodarone appears to be valuable in the treatment of ventricular and supraventricular arrhythmias, particularly those supraventricular arrythmias associated with Wolff-Parkinson-White syndrome, due to its effect on conduction in accessory pathways. Because of its toxicity however, should be reserved for patients resistant to conventional agents.

Class 4 antiarrhythmic agents

Calcium antagonists act by inhibiting the slow inward movement of calcium during phase 2 of depolarization. Verapamil and diltiazem are the only effective antiarrhythmics in this group because of their depressant effect on AV conduction. They are therefore of value in terminating supraventricular arrhythmias and AV nodal reentry tachycardias, including those associated with the Wolff-Parkinson-White syndrome. They also have a negative inotropic effect and cause peripheral vasodilatation. The latter compensates for the negative inotropic effect in patients with normal cardiac function, but in those with poor myocardial contractility heart failure may occur. Verapamil is completely absorbed after oral administration and undergoes marked and variable presystemic metabolism in the liver so that the bioavailability is only 10–20%. Its half-life is around 4 hours and so it has to be given thrice daily to protect against arrhythmias. Dosage should be reduced in hepatic impairment. It should be prescribed orally with β-blocking drugs only when the myocardium is relatively healthy and because of its effect on AV node conduction it cannot be used patients with severe sinus bradycardia or any degree of heart block. When it is administered intravenously, it should be given slowly with regular monitoring of the blood pressure, but should not be given by this route to patients already on beta blocker therapy.

ANTIANGINAL DRUGS

Angina pectoris is pain caused by myocardial ischaemia when myocardial oxygen demands outstrip supply. This can occur due to fixed stenosis in the coronary arteries due to atherosclerosis or more rarely due to acute spasm of the coronary arteries. Stable angina pectoris is generally related to exercise but other risk factors such as cigarette smoking, can aggravate the symptoms. Variant (or Prinzmetal) angina generally occurs with the patient at rest. In its pure form, the coronary arteries are angiographically normal, but develop intermittent spasm and this condition is rare. Spasm of the coronary arteries can coexist with fixed atherosclerotic occlusion however, and may contribute to the symptoms of angina at rest, nocturnal angina, exercise related angina and unstable angina. The aim of treatment is to restore the balance between myocardial oxygen consumption and supply and thus reduce the ischaemia.

Organic nitrates

Glyceryl trinitrate has been used for the treatment of angina pectoris for over 100 years and still remains the primary treatment for this condition. Organic nitrates act primarily by reducing cardiac preload by venous dilatation, resulting in reduced left ventricular size, wall tension and myocardial oxygen demand. Afterload may also be reduced due .to a slight fall in systemic vascular resistance and this may contribute to the relief of ischaemia. Finally there is some evidence that coronary artery dilatation can occur together with redistribution of coronary blood flow to ischaemic myocardium but the importance of this effect is still unknown. Glyceryl trinitrate is extensively metabolized on the first pass through the liver and is rapidly cleared by the body with a half-life of about 2 minutes. It is therefore necessary to give the drug by routes other than the oral route. Sublingual glyceryl trinitrate produces rapid symtomatic relief for about 20 to 30 minutes. Alternative approaches are to use an aerosal spray or transdermal preparation. The latter is especially useful for relief of angina at rest, particularly at night. Nitrates may also be used prophylactically before physical exertion or mental stress which would be expected to produce an anginal attack.

Isosorbide dinitrate. Isosorbide dinitrate has a longer half-life (45 minutes) and undergoes less presystemic metabolism so that it can be given by the oral route, although it must be administered at least 3 and perhaps 4 times daily. It is also effective after sublingual administration and although its effect comes on more slowly than glyceryl trinitrate it lasts longer. Sustained release preparations are also available. Both glyceryl trinitrate and isosorbide dinitrate can be given intravenously in emergency when pain is not relieved after other routes of administration. Isosorbide mononitrate is the active metabolite of isosorbide dinitrate, but it is not yet clear if it has any clinical advantages over the parent compound.

All organic nitrates cause flushing, headache, postural hypotension and reflex tachycardia. Methaemoglobinaemia due to oxidation of haemoglobin by nitrates is rare and most commonly seen with very large doses. Partial tolerance can also occur during chronic administration of the drug together with a possible exacerbation of angina on sudden withdrawal of the drug. Nitrates should therefore be gradually discontinued in those who have required large doses. As well as exerting beneficial effects in angina, nitrates may be useful in reducing preload in both acute left ventricular failure and chronic heart failure.

β-adrenergic blocking drugs

The major action of these drugs in angina pectoris is to reduce myocardial oxygen demand by reducing the sympathetic response to stresses (e.g. exercise). They are sometimes used as first-line agents in the prophylaxis of angina or as second-line agents when nitrates do not control symptoms. Sudden withdrawal of β-blockers can induce severe angina in a small proportion of patients, sometimes leading to myocardial infarction and it is important to gradually discontinue β-blockers when they are no longer indicated.

Calcium antagonists

Calcium antagonists relieve anginal pain by reducing myocardial oxygen consumption secondary to a decrease in afterload caused by arteriolar vasodilatation. They also appear to prevent coronary artery spasm in patients with variant angina and verapamil (but not nifedipine) appears to reduce cardiac output and thus may further reduce myocardial oxygen consumption. Calcium antagonists also have the advantage that unlike β-blockers they are not contraindicated in patients with obstructive airways disease.

Nifedipine is well absorbed after oral administration but undergoes high and variable presystemic metabolism. The half-life of elimination is about 4 hours and the drug is cleared by hepatic metabolism. Adverse effects of nifedipine are similar to those of nitrates, and headache, flushing and hypotension have been described. It can also cause peripheral oedema as a result of pre-capillarly vaso-dilatation, and painful erythema of the legs. Cardiac failure is often improved by the reduction in afterload caused by nifedipine.

Other agents

Perhexilene maleate reduces the frequency and severity of anginal attacks by an unknown mechanism. It does not appear to precipitate heart failure or bronchospasm, but other unwanted effects are common and include abnormalities in liver function tests and peripheral neuropathy. There is evidence that adverse effects of the drug are commoner in the 10% of the population who are slow oxidisers of perhexiline (page 20).

HYPOLIPIDAEMIC AGENTS

The association of atherosclerosis and ischaemic heart disease with high blood levels of cholesterol has led to the introduction of drugs to lower cholesterol. The relationship between hypertriglyceridaemia and ischaemic heart disease is less clear but severe hypertriglyceridaemia can lead to episodes of pancreatitis and should therefore be controlled.

Initial treatment should be with diet which achieves and maintains the ideal body weight. Saturated animal fats and cholesterol should be reduced and replaced with unsaturated (e.g. vegetable) fat. Those who fail to response to dietary measures should be considered for drug therapy.

Cholestyramine and colestipol hydrochloride are bile acid binding resins which lower plasma cholesterol by reducing absorption from the gut, although they may occasionally cause triglyceride levels to rise. They often cause abdominal discomfort, heartburn and flatulence, and may prevent absorbtion of fat soluble vitamins and drugs (e.g. warfarin or thyroxine). Recent work has indicated for the first time that reduction in excessively raised cholesterol by diet and cholestyramine reduces cardiovascular mortality and morbidity.

Nicotinic acid. Nicotinic acid lowers plasma cholesterol and triglycerides. Although the mechanism of action is not clear, it may be related at least in part to decreased hepatic synthesis of lipoproteins. Adverse effects include flushing and pruritis which may improve on continued therapy. The drug can also cause vomiting, diarrhoea and dyspepsia and rarely peptic ulceration. Plasma urate and blood glucose may also rise and the drug should be used with caution in patients with diabetes or gout. Nicofuranose is an analogue of nicotinic acid which is slowly hydrolysed to the latter agent. It has similar actions but may be better tolerated.

Clofibrate and bezafibrate. Both drugs reduce plasma cholesterol and triglycerides by reducing hepatic secretion of lipoproteins. They tend to be reserved for patients with severe hypertriglycerid-aemia. As well as gastrointestinal adverse effects, they can rarely cause a myositis-like syndrome, particularly in those with renal impairment.

Probucol. Probucol is a compound unrelated to the other agents. It appears to act by enhancing removal of LDL lipoprotein from the circulation, thus lowering plasma cholesterol. Like the other agents, it can cause gastrointestinal symptoms, and very rarely angioneurotic oedema or hypersensitivity reactions.

FURTHER READING

Opie L H 1980 Drugs and the heart. Lancet

9

Prostaglandins, platelets and clotting

PROSTAGLANDINS

Prostaglandin was the name originally given to a lipid substance, derived from human seminal plasma, which contracted smooth muscle. Substances with similar activity were found in seminal fluid in other animals, and in extracts of prostate and the vesicular glands. Today the term prostaglandin refers to a large family of closely related long chain unsaturated fatty acids, all derivatives of arachidonic acid (Fig. 9.1). They were originally identified by alphabetical and numeral subscripts but those in clinical use have now been given approved names. Under suitable conditions, a large number of tissues can be induced to release prostaglandins into the circulation, but their contribution to pharmacological and physiological activity has not been fully elucidated.

Prostaglandins of the E and F series appear to be associated with inflammatory reactions. They also have a role in stimulating the uterine smooth muscle during labour and perhaps during conception. They have been used therapeutically to induce labour and abortion as well as to promote cervical ripening. Appreciable quantities of prostaglandins are present in brain tissue, and micro-injection techniques have shown stimulatory and inhibitory action on neurones in the central nervous system. They may, therefore, have a direct or indirect role in central nervous transmission.

Various prostaglandins have been shown to have vasoconstrictor, vasodilator, broncho-constrictor and bronchodilator activity and some of the prostaglandins of the E series can decrease gastric acid production. This chapter is concerned with those prostaglandins having activity either on vascular tone or on platelet aggregation.

Epoprostenol

This prostaglandin (originally called PGI2 or prostacyclin) was discovered in 1976. It is synthesized from arachidonic acid in the

157

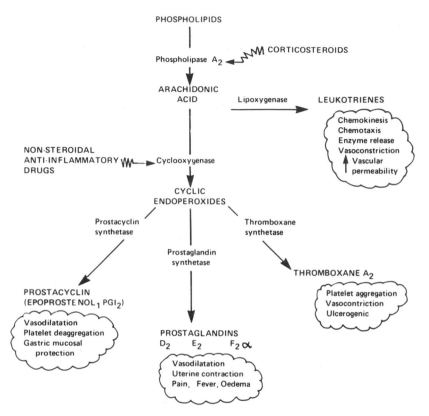

Fig. 9.1 Synthesis of prostaglandins.

arterial intima and is a potent vascular smooth muscle relaxant and inhibitor of platelet aggregation. It has opposing effects to the prostaglandin produced by the platelet (thromboxane A2) and it has been suggested that these two substances play a natural role in maintaining the integrity of the vascular endothelium. When the vascular endothelium is damaged platelets can plug the breach since their aggregation (induced by thromboxane A2) is no longer antagonized. Epoprostenol has a biological half-life of 2 to 3 minutes. It is rapidly hydrolysed to an inactive metabolite (6 keto PGFI α) and its normal circulating level in man is well below that necessary to produce pharmacological effects. It must, therefore, be given in large doses by continuous intravenous infusion.

The therapeutic effects of epoprostenol are related to inhibitory effects on platelet aggregation which has been stimulated by artificial surfaces in extracorporial circulations. Platelet aggregation under these circumstances can lead to thrombocytopaenia and bleeding, as well as to microaggregates which may cause systemic emboli. The neurological sequelae that can follow cardiopulmonary bypass are probably related to this phenomenon occurring in the arterial tree. Although epoprostenol may reduce the degree of platelet loss in extracorporeal circulations, it has not yet been shown to reduce the incidence of neurological sequelae after cardiopulmonary bypass. In haemodialysis it can partially or completely replace the use of heparin, but it is very much more expensive at present. Early evidence indicates that it may improve survival in patients with fulminant hepatic failure who are treated by charcoal haemoperfusion, since by reducing the platelet loss it allows the haemoperfusion to be continued for longer periods.

Alprostadil. Formerly known as Prostaglandin E1, this agent relaxes vascular smooth muscle and has a slight antiaggregatory effect on platelets. It is metabolized rapidly by pulmonary capillary endothelium so that its half-life is less than 2 minutes. Like epoprostenol, therefore, it must be given by continuous intravenous infusion. Its only clinical indication at present is to maintain patency of the ductus arteriosus in cyanotic congenital heart disease, improving pulmonary blood flow until the cardiac defect can be surgically repaired. Conversely, indomethacin and other non-steroidal anti-inflammatory drugs have been used to promote closure of the ductus in circumstances where this is clinically valuable. Adverse effects of alprostadil include fever, apnoea and convulsions and possibly weakening of the wall of the ductus arteriosus after prolonged use.

Drugs modifying prostaglandin metabolism

At least part of the inflammatory action of steroids is mediated through their inhibition of phospholipase A, (Fig. 9.1) the enzyme which mediates the production of arachidonic acid from phospholipids. Inhibitors of the enzyme mediating the next step of the production of prostaglandins, cyclooxygenase, include aspirin and the other non-steroidal anti-inflammatory agents. Aspirin irreversibly acetylates the platelet enzyme cyclo-oxygenase (Fig. 9.1), thereby preventing the formation of thromboxane A2. In conventional doses it also irreversibly inhibits the same enzyme in the blood vessel wall and blocks the formation of prostacyclin. Lower doses of aspirin may selectively spare the vessel wall enzyme leaving a predominantly deaggretory effect. Studies are under way to examine the therapeutic implications of this in diseases of the arterial tree in which thrombosis plays an important role. Work is also being performed on production of more selective inhibitors of thromboxane synthetase.

Sulphinpyrazone is also a competitive inhibitor of cyclo-oxygenase and it has been used to maintain graft patency after coronary artery bypass grafting. Although one study showed it to be useful in secondary prevention of mortality after myocardial infarction, criticisms of the design and analysis of the study have resulted in it being little used for this indication at present.

Dipyridamole is a vasodilator which has phosphodiesterase inhibitory activity. This leads to an increase in platelet cyclic AMP and subsequent inhibition of aggregation, not mediated by the prostaglandin pathway. It has been used in conjunction with anticoagulants to prevent thrombus formation on prosthetic heart valves. Because of its vasodilator activity it can cause headache, flushing and hypotension.

ANTICOAGULANTS

Anticoagulant drugs inhibit the clotting mechanism (Fig. 9.2), but they have no effect on platelet aggregation which initiates subsequent clotting especially in the arterial tree. They are therefore of more value in venous than in arterial thrombosis.

Oral anticoagulants

Oral anticoagulants are either derivatives of 4-hydroxy-coumarin or of indane-1,3,dione. Coumarins were first discovered in improperly cured sweetclover which caused haemorrhagic disease in cattle. Warfarin is the most widely used agent and none of the other coumarins (e.g. dicoumarol) have any advantages over it. Warfarin like all coumarins, antagonises the physiological function of Vitamin K, a co-factor in the synthesis of clotting factors II, VII, IX and X (the Vitamin K dependent clotting factors). Coumarins act on Vitamin K by inhibiting the Vitamin K dependent carboxylation of glutamyl residues on the clotting factor precursors so that they do not have calcium binding sites and are therefore inactive. The onset of anticoagulant activity is primarily dependent on the half-lives of the Vitamin K dependent clotting factors, principally Factor VII, which has a half-life of 1.5–6 hours.

Warfarin is rapidly and completely absorbed after oral adminis-

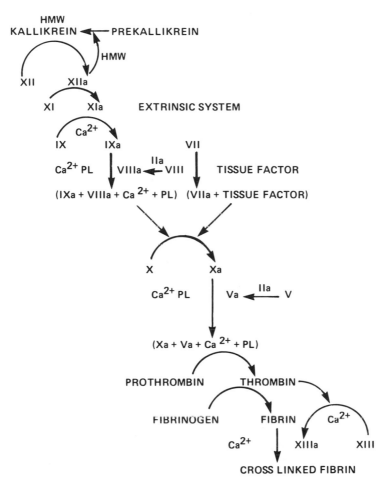

Fig. 9.2 Cascade mechanism of blood coagulation. PL : phospholipid;
CA^{2+} : calcium ion; HMW : high molecular weight kininogen (reproduced with
permission from Poller L 1981. Recent advances in blood coagulation. Churchill
Livingstone, Edinburgh).

tration. It is highly bound to plasma albumin and has a small distribution volume of 7 litres. Small amounts do cross the placenta,
however, and since it is teratogenic, it should not be used in pregnancy. It does not enter breast milk in quantities sufficient to
produce anticoagulation in the fetus. It is completely metabolized
by the liver with a half-life of 36 to 50 hours, and although some

of the metabolites have anticoagulant activity they are probably of little importance.

The main indications for oral anticoagulants are the treatment and prevention of deep vein thrombosis and pulmonary embolus. They are also used to prevent thrombo-embolism from diseased or prosthetic heart valves. The major adverse effect of warfarin is bleeding, the risk of which is directly proportional to the degree of anticoagulation. Anticoagulant effect is measured using the ratio between the one-stage prothrombin time of the patient's plasma and that of a control subject, using British Comparative Thromboplastin (BCR). Patients with thrombosis in the arterial circulation usually require a BCR between 3 to 4 for adequate protection, whereas those with venous thrombosis are adequately protected with a BCR between 2 and 3. The drug is normally started using an induction dose of 10 mg which can be adjusted according to the BCR, measured initially daily. The daily maintenance dose is usually 2–8 mg. The elderly and patients with heart failure or liver disease are particularly sensitive to warfarin. Skin necrosis occurs very rarely in susceptible subjects when the drug is first started. The antidote for warfarin is Vitamin K which can be given intravenously or orally, depending on the clinical situation. It is variably absorbed after oral administration and a more consistent response is obtained after using the intravenous route. Rapid intravenous administration of Vitamin K can be associated with severe adverse effects however. If continued anticoagulant control is necessary only small doses of Vitamin K should be given (e.g. 1 mg intravenously) and reversal of the anticoagulation occurs in approximately 24 hours. Complete reversal may require larger doses (10–20 mg daily) over several days because of the long half-life of warfarin relative to Vitamin K. In emergency, immediate reversal may be obtained using fresh protein plasma.

Numerous drugs have been shown to interact with warfarin. Enzyme inducing drugs such as rifampicin and the barbiturates decrease anticoagulant effect because they enhance warfarin metabolism. Other agents inhibit warfarin metabolism (e.g. mefenamic acid, azapropazone, metronidazole and cimetidine). The possibility of drug interaction should always therefore be kept in mind when any change in drug therapy is considered. Patients on warfarin should never be given intramuscular injections because of the risks of haematoma formation.

Phenindione is an alternative (indanedione) agent which has a higher incidence of adverse effects, including skin rash, agranulocytosis, diarrhoea, renal and liver damage. It also enters breast milk in significant quantities and is now rarely used.

Heparin.

Heparin is a complex mucopolysaccharide, occuring naturally in mast cells. It is the strongest organic acid in the body and exerts its anticoagulant effect by accelerating the rate at which anti-thrombin III (an α-2 globulin) neutralizes the activated clotting factors in the intrinsic pathway of the coagulation cascade (Fig. 9.2). It is not absorbed orally and is given either intravenously or subcutaneously. It is metabolized rapidly with a half-life of 1 to 2 hours and clearance is increased in patients with pulmonary embolism. It does not cross the placenta or enter breast milk. The most common adverse effect is haemorrage which is reduced by giving the drug by continuous infusion (rather than by intermittent intravenous injection) and by monitoring the degree of anticoagulation using a derivative of the active partial thromboplastin time such as the Kaolin Cephalin clotting time (KCCT). This should be kept between 1.5 and 2.5 × control plasma. Since the KCCT ratio is exponentially related to the heparin infusion rate, smaller increments in unfusion rate are needed as the KCCT approaches the therapeutic range. Elderly women seem to be particularly predisposed to haemorrhage.

Thrombocytopaenia is a rather uncommon adverse effect. Osteoporosis and alopecia are also rare and usually associated with prolonged therapy. Interactions with heparin are unusual unless the drugs are added to the intravenous bottle containing the drug. Like warfarin, it should never be given by intramuscular injection. Protamine sulphate is a direct antagonist of heparin and 1 mg neutralizes 100 units of heparin when given within 15 minutes. If given in excess, protamine itself can produce an anticoagulant effect.

Fibrinolytic and antifibrinolytic drugs

A fibrinolytic mechanism is normally responsible for lysing small clots which occur within the vascular system. A plasminogen activator (Fig. 9.3) is released by the vascular endothelium, and the enzyme which is formed, plasmin, acts on fibrin and fibrinogen to produce soluble derivatives. Plasminogen activators, (e.g. streptokinase and urokinase) can be administered intravenously and

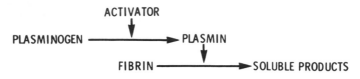

Fig. 9.3 The fibrinolytic mechanism.

produce the same effect as endogenous activators. In contrast to anticoagulant drugs, fibrinolytic compounds can dissolve established clots, (e.g. in deep vein thrombosis and pulmonary embolism) as well as preventing further formation. Although best given by infusion through a catheter whose tip lies close to the clot, this is not often possible and the drug is then given by intravenous infusion. A loading dose is given, followed by a maintenance dose for 48–72 hours. The dose is adjusted according to the thrombin clotting time.

Streptokinase is derived from β-haemolytic streptococci. It is highly antigenic and is liable to be inactivated by circulating IgG antibodies from previous streptococcal infections. A loading dose of 250 000 units is sufficient to neutralize the antibody and provide an excess for fibrinolysis. Immediate allergic reactions and pyrexia are so common that it is usual to give prophylactic steroid therapy before the infusion. Urokinase is derived from human kidney-cell cultures or normal urine, and is non-antigenic. It is extremely expensive.

The main risk is of haemorrhage, and an antifibrinolysin (antiplasmin) such as epsilon aminocaproic acid or tranexamic acid should be available. Antiplasmins are also used in conditions associated with high circulating levels of plasmin (e.g. in concealed or accidental haemorrhage in obstetrics, or following handling of the lungs during surgery). Aprotinin has antitrypsin as well as antiplasmin and antikinin properties, and is used in the treatment of acute pancreatitis, although its value is uncertain.

10

Diuretics

A diuretic is a drug which increases the volume of urine produced by the kidney. It may produce its effects in one of two ways:
1. By increasing renal blood flow and glomerular filtration rate.
2. By inhibiting the reabsorption of sodium by the renal tubule.

Drugs which increase renal blood flow

Digitalis glycosides. Cardiac glycosides, such as digoxin, which increase the output of the failing heart and so increase renal perfusion and glomerular filtration, may be said to have diuretic activity. In addition, digoxin has been shown to have a direct action on the renal tubule to inhibit sodium reabsorption, but whether this is important in therapeutic doses is uncertain.

Xanthines (see also p. 173). It has long been known that coffee, tea and other related beverages have a diuretic action. This is due to the xanthine drugs caffeine, theobromine and theophylline which they contain. These, together with others such as aminophylline, inhibit the enzyme phosphodiesterase. They increase renal blood flow by increasing the force of cardiac contraction and hence the cardiac output where this is reduced, and by dilating renal medullary blood vessels. They may also directly inhibit sodium reabsorption by the renal tubules. Aminophylline is the most important of this group of drugs in clinical use, and is usually administered by slow intravenous injection.

Drugs which inhibit sodium reabsorption

Fluid retention is usually due to a primary retention of sodium in the body, and the most effective way to reduce excess body water is to increase sodium excretion by the kidneys. It is necessary to induce a state of negative sodium balance in which the quantity of sodium lost by the body is in excess of that taken in.

Sodium reabsorption occurs throughout the length of the renal tubule. The greatest part of the filtered load, between 60 and 70%, is reabsorbed together with water in the proximal part of the tubule. In the ascending limb of the loop of Henle sodium is actively reabsorbed without water, leading to hypertonicity of the surrounding medullary tissue, and hypotonic fluid passes into the distal tubule. Here, under the influence of aldosterone, sodium is exchanged for potassium, and so an increase in the sodium load in the distal part of the distal tubule is associated with increased exchange leading to potassium loss. As the hypotonic filtrate then passes down the collecting tubules through the hypertonic medullary tissue, water is reabsorbed under the control of antidiuretic hormone.

Thiazides. This group of diuretic agents was developed as the result of a search for more potent carbonic anhydrase inhibitors, although in fact, they owe but little of their action to this effect. Their site of action is uncertain, but probably involves inhibition of sodium reabsorption in the proximal part of the distal tubule. Although they are weaker than the mercurial diuretics (e.g. mersalyl), they have the advantage of being effective after oral administration, and some preparations can be given intravenously. A large number of these compounds are now available including bendrofluazide, chlorothiazide, cyclopenthiazide, hydrocholorothiazide, hydroflumethiazide and polythiazide. Although chemically distinct from the thiazides, chlorthalidone, indapamide and xipamide closely resemble them in their pharmacological and adverse effects. It is unlikely that one is superior to another, however, in terms of therapeutic effectiveness or lack of adverse effects, and all show the following features:

1. Potassium loss. The increased sodium load reaching the distal part of the distal tubule results in an increased exchange of sodium for potassium under the influence of aldosterone. If a marked diuresis occurs with depletion of the blood volume, aldosterone secretion increases leading to an even greater sodium–potassium exchange and potassium loss. Potassium supplements or potassium sparing diuretics (see below) should be given, therefore, to patients receiving regular thiazide treatment for a long period.

2. Hyperglycaemia may occur in patients treated with thiazide drugs, with increased insulin requirements in diabetic patients. The mechanism of this effect isnot known.

3. Hyperuricaemia frequently occurs, with attacks of clinical gout in patients with a previous history of the condition. This is probably due to a reduction in uric acid excretion by the kidney

together with contraction of the extracellular fluid volume. Tienilic acid has potentially useful uric-acid excreting and hypouricaemic properties together with diuretic activity. Unfortunately it has been withdrawn from clinical trial because of reports of liver toxicity.

4. Hypotensive effects (see p. 71).

5. Decrease in urinary calcium excretion. Thiazides are used in management of idiopathic hypercalcuria associated with recurrent renal calculi. Urinary calcium excretion may be reduced by as much as 40%, while serum calcium concentrations may increase slightly.

6. Reduction in urine volume in patients with nephrogenic diabetes insipidus (see page 202).

Bumetanide and frusemide. These are related chemically to, but are very much more potent than, the thiazide diuretics. They appear to inhibit sodium reabsorption in the proximal part of the distal tubule, but also have a marked action on the ascending limb of the loop of Henle. They are therefore called 'loop' or 'high-potency' diuretics. For an equivalent degree of diuresis they produce less potassium loss than the thiazides, but when they are used in larger doses for a powerful diuresis the loss of potassium is considerable and supplementary potassium must be given to patients receiving regular treatment. Excessive sodium and chloride diuresis can lead to severe blood volume depletion, hypotension and uraemia. Like the thiazides they have hyperglycaemic, hyperuricaemic and hypotensive effects. They may be given orally or intravenously, the latter route being particularly appropriate for use in emergencies such as pulmonary oedema. They may be used intravenously alone or together with a thiazide diuretic, to increase calcium excretion in patients with hypercalcaemia.

Ethacrynic acid. This drug is of the same order of potency as bumetanide and frusemide, exerting its effect like the latter predominantly on the ascending limb of the loop of Henle and the proximal part of the distal tubule. Its complications and adverse effects are similar with the addition of transient deafness possibly due to interference with the production of perilymph in the inner ear. Its use should be restricted to acute emergencies, in which it may be administered by cautious intravenous injection.

Spironolactone. This drug is a synthetic steroid, in structure resembling aldosterone, of which it is a competitive antagonist. It is, therefore, inactive in adrenalectomized patients and its effects are limited in physiological states in which aldosterone secretion is reduced to a minimum. It inhibits the exchange of sodium for potassium ions in the distal part of the distal tubule which is under the control of aldosterone. As the sodium reabsorption here accounts for only a small part of that in the renal tubule as a whole, the diuretic activity of spironolactone is weak. It is most effective in those conditions in which there are high circulating levels of aldosterone, for example, hepatic cirrhosis and the nephrotic syndrome. When given together with diuretics acting at more proximal sites in the nephron, such as the thiazides, it reduces the potassium loss which they produce as well as increasing sodium excretion. It may still be necessary to give potassium supplements, however. Like the thiazides, spironolactone causes a moderate fall in blood pressure by itself, and potentiates the action of other antihypertensive drugs. Toxic effects include headache, nausea and vomiting, menstrual abnormalities, hirsutism and impotence. Tender nipples or painful gynaecomastia may occur, particularly in men. Hyperkalaemia may occur in patients with renal impairment.

Triamterene. Triamterene is a pteridine derivative chemically related to inhibitors of folic acid synthesis, but with important diuretic activity. Although it inhibits the exchange of sodium for potassium in the distal tubule, this is independent of aldosterone antagonism, and occurs even in the adrenalectomized animal. Like spironolactone, it is a relatively weak diuretic, but is useful in combination with the thiazides where it potentiates the sodium excreting effect and reduces potassium loss. It is especially useful in those conditions, such as hepatic ascites, where hypokalaemia is particularly dangerous. In fact, hyperkalaemia may occur when it is used alone. It sometimes produces nausea, vomiting and diarrhoea.

Amiloride. This drug resembles triameterene in its structure, pharmacology, therapeutic indications and adverse effects. When given with thiazide diuretics it potentiates sodium excretion and reduces potassium loss. Excessive sodium and water loss may lead to an increase in blood urea and vascular collapse. Dangerous hyperkalaemia can occur.

Carbonic anhydrase inhibitors. In the proximal and distal tubules sodium ions are exchanged for hydrogen ions generated from H_2O and CO_2 under the influence of the enzyme carbonic anhydrase. Inhibition of this enzyme with drugs such as acetazolamide reduces the availability of hydrogen ions and so leads to an increase in excretion of sodium together with bicarbonate with the production of an alkaline urine. The increase in bicarbonate excretion leads to a metabolic acidosis which in turn reduces the effectiveness of the drug. The action of acetazolamide may disappear therefore, after only 48 hours of treatment. For this reason it has been largely superseded by the thiazides and other diuretics. Toxic effects include drowsiness, mental confusion and paraesthesiae of the extremities.

Important interactions of diuretics

1. *Lithium.* Thiazides indirectly increase reabsorption of lithium in the renal tubule leading to the risk of lithium toxicity.
2. *Non-steroidal anti-inflammatory drugs.* Aspirin, indomethacin and other drugs of this type antagonise the diuretic and hypotensive actions of thiazides and loop diuretics. The mechanism of this interaction is not completely understood but may involve inhibition of prostaglandin synthesis or be due to the salt retention produced by these anti-inflammatory drugs.
3. *Antibiotic nephrotoxicity and ototoxicity* induced, for example by aminoglycosides and cephaloridine, may be enhanced by frusemide.
4. *Hypokalaemia-inducing steroids.* The risk of hypokalaemia is greatly increased if thiazides or loop diuretics are used in patients receiving corticosteroids or carbenoxolone (pages 40, 183).

Osmotic diuretics

Active sodium reabsorption in the proximal tubule is accompanied by absorption of isosmotic amounts of water. The administration of an osmotic diuretic and its presence in the lumen of the renal tubule opposes this reabsorption of water and, indirectly, reduces sodium reabsorption. Apart from this action, some of the osmotic diuretics such as mannitol, also improve renal perfusion.

Mannitol, a non-metabolized sugar alcohol, is the most important of this group of agents. It is administered intravenously in concentrations of 5 to 20% and is freely filtered at the glomerulus. It is not reabsorbed by the tubules, and so has been used to measure the glomerular filtration rate. The infusion must be carefully monitored as it may lead to increased circulating volume and central venous pressure, cardiac failure, plasma hyperosmolality and hyponataemia. Indications for treatment with mannitol are:

(a) Oedema refractory to other diuretics given alone or in combination. In such cases it may initiate a diuresis which is then maintained by other agents.

(b) Drug poisoning where a forced diuresis increases the rate of elimimation.

(c) To improve renal blood flow in conditions where renal failure might occur, such as shock and in cadiovascular surgery.

Potassium supplements

Although potassium loss may lead to a severe degree of hypokalaemia with its associated muscle weakness, mental disturbances, cardiac effects, and, in patients with hepatic ascites, risk of encephalopathy, the true risk of this happening as a result of diuretic treatment is controversial. There is no doubt about its importance in patients receiving digitalis for heart disease, in whom hypokalaemia increases the risk of digitalis intoxication. It is also more likely to occur in the elderly, particularly those with poor dietary habits. In general, however, the risks to a patient from hyperkalaemia are greater than those from hypokalaemia, except in patients receiving digitalis, and the routine use of potassium supplements wherever a thiazide-type or loop diuretic is being used is clinically unwise. Potassium loss associated with use of these diuretics may be reduced by combined treatment with a potassium sparing diuretic such as spironolactone, triamterene or amiloride. However, these drugs carry the hazard of hyperkalaemia particularly when potassium supplements are also given. In hypertension the addition of a β-adrenoceptor blocking drug (page 67) or captopril (page 73) will often reduce the potassium loss sufficient to render potassium supplementation or the addition of a potassium sparing diuretic unnecessary.

When treatment with potassium supplements is indicated, potassium chloride is the compound of choice since chloride is required to correct the alkalosis that accompanies the hypokalaemia. In solution potassium chloride is poorly tolerated because of its nauseous effects, and other formulations have therefore been introduced which are better tolerated. Slow-release preparations, in which potassium chloride diffuses out of a wax matrix as it passes through the small intestine, appear to be relatively safe compared with earlier enteric-coated formulations which were associated with hazards of small bowel necrosis, ulceration, perforation and stricture. An effervescent preparation containing betaine hydrochloride and potassium bicarbonate is available and appears to be well tolerated and effective.

The normal diet contains about 80–100 mEq daily of potassium.

Slow release preparations such as Slow-K contain about 8 mEq potassium, so that 10 daily would be required to provide this intake, although such doses are seldom used. Clinical hypokalaemia probably requires doses in excess of 60–80 mEq daily, and it may then be more convenient to use 10% potassium chloride elixir because of its rapid absorption from the stomach. Daily oral doses in excess of 100 mEq should only be administered with great caution because of the cardiac risks of hyperkalaemia.

Intravenous administration of potassium chloride should only be carried out slowly under constant supervision for evidence of cardiac dysrhythmias. It should not exceed a rate of 20 mmol per hour or a concentration of 50 mmol per litre.

11

Drugs and the respiratory system

Respiratory centre

Stimulation. There is a variety of compounds which stimulate the respiratory and cardiovascular centres in the midbrain and hypothalamus. They were widely used to stimulate respiration in patients with respiratory depression due to drugs or disease, but with the development of mechanical devices for artificial ventilation they are now seldom employed. Their therapeutic ratio is generally low, and overdosage induces convulsions and delirium. Among the more important of these compounds are pentylenetetrazol, bemegride, nikethamide, doxapram and picrotoxin. Almitrine, at present undergoing clinical investigation, appears to stimulate respiration by a peripheral action, probably involving the carotid body.

Depression. A wide range of central nervous depressant drugs produce respiratory depression when administered in excess of their therapeutic doses, including barbiturates, alcohol and the narcotic analgesic drugs.

Drugs and the bronchus

The pharmacology of bronchial smooth muscle is summarized in Table 11.1.

Bronchospastic drugs

Bronchoconstriction may be produced by acetylcholine, muscarine, histamine, 5-hydroxytryptamine, bradykinin and slow-reacting substance (SRS) all of which produce spasm of bronchial smooth muscle. There is also evidence that some prostaglandins may posses bronchoconstrictor and some bronchodilator properties. The role of one or more of these pharmacological agents in bronchial asthma is still uncertain.

Table 11.1   Pharmacology of bronchial muscle

	Constriction	Dilatation
Neurogenic		
Parasympathetic	+	
Sympathetic		+
Autonomic receptor		
Cholinergic	+	
Adrenergic α	+	
β₂		+
Histamine	+	
5-Hydroxytryptamine	+	
Others		
Kinins	+	
SRS-A	+	
Prostaglandins	+	+

β-Adrenoceptor blocking drugs may produce bronchoconstriction by preventing sympathetically mediated bronchodilator tone (p. 65).

Bronchodilators

Sympathomimetic amines. Sympathetic stimulation produces bronchodilatation through β-receptor activity, and therefore β-receptor agonists such as isoprenaline and orciprenaline are potent bronchodilators compared with noradrenaline which primarily activates α-adrenergic receptors. Adrenaline, which has marked affinity for both α- and β-receptors, is also a potent bronchodilator drug. These drugs stimulate β-receptors generally and therefore increase the rate and force of cardiac contraction in doses which dilate the bronchi.

Selective β₂-receptor agonists such as isoetharine, salbutamol, rimiterol, fenoterol and reproterol dilate the bronchi and reduce the bronchoconstrictor effects of histamine and acetylcholine in doses which to not produce any cardiac effects. Higher doses, however, do produce cardiac stimulation and tremor, and these drugs should therefore be used with caution in patients with underlying heart disease. Although some may be administered orally and parenterally, the most convenient route is by inhalation from fixed dose aerosol dispensers and fewer adverse effects occur with this route of administration. The bronchodilator action appears rapidly within minutes of inhalation and may persist for some hours.

Xanthines. These drugs act by inhibiting phosphodiesterase and hence have actions which resemble sympathetic stimulation, but are not blocked by adrenergic neurone or receptor blocking drugs. Aminophylline, which is a combination of theophylline and ethylenediamine, has useful bronchodilator properties in conditions such as bronchial asthma and pulmonary oedema where bronchoconstriction is present. It can be given intravenously in status asthmaticus, but slow administration is necessary because of the danger of cardiac dysrhythmias and fits. By suppository it is erratically absorbed. Theophylline and aminophylline are now available in slow release oral preparations which produce sustained therapeutic plasma levels for up to 10–12 hours and need only to be administered every 12 hours. They should replace older preparations such as choline theophyllinate which produce adequate plasma levels for only a few hours and have a higher incidence of gastric irritation. Other xanthine bronchodilator drugs include acepifylline, diprophylline and etamiphylline.

Anticholinergic drugs. Drugs which block the muscarinic actions of acetylcholine, such as atropine, have bronchodilator properties, and the increase in airway resistance produced in asthmatic and bronchitic patients by aerosols of histamine or carbon dust is abolished by the administration of atropine methonitrate. It is, therefore, included in some aerosol preparations with sympathomimetic amines. Although its bronchodilator action may be an advantage, it also reduces the volume of secretions in the bronchial tree, resulting in decreased fluidity and increased viscosity. The secretions may then be more difficult to expectorate, leading to obstructed airflow and pulmonary infection. These effects may more than overweigh any advantage gained by using atropine in bronchial asthma.

Deptropine and ipratropium are other anticholinergic drugs which are probably less effective than the β-receptor agonists such as salbutamol in asthma, but appear to be as effective in patients with chronic bronchitis who have reversible airways obstruction. Effects on sputum viscosity appear to be unimportant.

Disodium cromoglycate

This drug is not a bronchodilator, nor does it antagonize mediators of tissue reaction such as histamine or slow-reacting substance. Its main action is prophylactic, reducing the incidence and severity of allergic asthmatic attacks, and the dosage of corticosteroids and bronchodilator drugs required by asthmatic patients. Its value in the treatment of acute attacks is not well established. The mechanism of its action is uncertain, but it may involve inhibition of release of histamine and slow-reacting substance from the mast cells by stabilization of the mast cell membrane, so preventing exocytosis (p. 50).

Disodium cromoglycate is a powder, poorly absorbed from the gut. It is, therefore, administered by inhalation from a special dispenser, a spinhaler, in which a propeller activated by suction creates a cloud of powder from the punctured capsule in which it is contained. Isoprenaline is included in some preparations to protect against bronchospasm caused by inhalation of a dry powder. It may also be of value in other conditions with an allergic basis, such as hay fever, allergic conjuncitives, aphthous ulceration and lactose intolerance.

Ketotifen

Ketotifen combines antihistamine with anti-allergic properties similar to those of disodium cromoglycate, but has the advantage that it is active after oral ingestion. Its role in management of asthma and other allergic conditions is being assessed. Its most common adverse effect is sedation which can occur even at therapeutic doses.

Bronchial asthma

Bronchial asthma has three principal components, increased tone of the smooth muscle within the bronchial walls, increased vascular engorgement of the submucosal tissues, and increased secretion by mucosal glands. These factors may be produced experimentally by a variety of substances such as histamine, slow-reacting substance of anaphylaxis (SRA-A) and 5-hydroxytryptamine, some of which may be responsible in part for allergic forms of the condition. These mediators are released from mast cells in response to antigen-antibody interaction on the cell surface. It is probable that this release is inhibited to some extent by stimulation of β-receptors on the mast cell membrane which leads to an increase in intracellular cyclic AMP (page 53). Parasympathetic activity mediated by release of acetylcholine, also produces increased tone and secretion, and may be responsible for asthmatic attacks triggered by psychogenic stimuli.

Prophylaxis. The incidence and severity of attacks may be reduced by regular administration of (a) disodium cromoglycate or ketotifen which interfere with the allergic response, (b) bronchodilator drugs such as the sympathomimetic amines ephedrine given orally, orciprenaline given orally or by aerosol, and salbutamol given orally or by aerosol. Xanthines such as theophylline and its derivatives may be given orally. Adjusting the dose to produce a serum level of 40 to 100 μmol/1 (9 to 18 μg/ml) has been shown to give an optimum bronchodilator effect; (c) corticosteroids. Oral treatment with prednisolone or other corticosteroids is often effective, but is associated with the risk of adrenal suppression with its ensuing complications (p. 228). Beclomethasone and betamethasone are administered by aerosol and have been shown to have prophylactic value, without producing significant adrenal suppression in usual therapeutic doses. They may, however, be associated with fungal infections of the trachea and bronchi.

Treatment of acute attack. While some authorities still advocate the use of subcutaneous adrenaline in the acute asthmatic attack, it is now becoming accepted practice to begin treatment in hospital with inhaled salbutamol administered through a ventilator such as the Bird model. Amniophylline may be given very slowly over 10 to 15 minutes by intravenous injection or by infusion, with continuous monitoring of the heart rate. Intravenous hydrocortisone in high doses is also given followed by oral prednisolone, again in high dosage. Oxygen should be given. If facilities for arterial blood gas estimations are available and there is no history of chronic obstructive airway disease, a high inspired oxygen concentration is both safe and desirable. In other circumstances, however, a concentration not exceeding 35% should be administered, because arterial carbon dioxide concentrations may rise steeply in some asthmatic patients, particularly children. A marked respiratory acidosis is often found in severe asthmatic attacks, and this may contribute to resistance to the bronchodilator action of sympathomimetic drugs such as salbutamol. It is important, therefore, to correct any acid-base disturbance which occurs. If the patient does not respond satisfactorily to these measures, intubation, or even tracheostomy, with assisted or controlled ventilation should be considered.

Dangers of excessive aerosal usage. Following reports of an increase in the number of children dying from asthma in Great Britain between 1960 and 1965, it was suggested that this might be associated with excessive use of sympathomimetic agents in the form of metered or pressurized aerosols of isoprenaline, orciprenaline or adrenaline. A comprehensive analysis has demonstrated a marked correlation between sales and prescriptions of these formulations over the years 1960 to 1967 and deaths from asthma, and has also shown that as the sale of pressurized aerosols began to fall from 1966, so the mortality curve has shown a sharp decline. Althoughthe sympathomimetic amines might be considered to be the most likely agents responsible for the toxicity of these preparations in view of their known cardiotoxic effects, the possibility must be considered that the fluorinated methane and ethane derivatives which are commonly used as aerosol propellants may play a part. There have been reports of deaths in young people who inhaled these fluorocarbons for their central stimulant effects, and it has been suggested that these substances can sensitize the myocardium to circulating catecholamines during hypoxia and produce a cardiac dysrthythmia. Estimations of these propellants, however, from chronic overusers of such bronchodilator aerosols have shown that the blood levels reached are probably not high enough to produce such myocardial sensitization. It seems probable that many of the deaths occurring in the 1960s, and indeed that still occur, resulted from complacency on the part of patients, relatives and doctors because of an unwarranted confidence in the new sympathomimetic drugs, and from inadequate management, particularly in the use of steroids.

Expectorants

Expectorants are used in inflammatory conditions of the respiratory tract and are claimed to increase the volume of bronchial secretion, and render it less tenacious. In general they are emetic compounds administered in subemetic doses, emesis being preceded by increased activity of secretory glands. The most commonly used are standard formulations of sodium chloride, ipecacuanha, ammonium chloride, potassium iodide, and squill. They are relatively harmless in standard doses, although chronic ingestion of potassium iodide by patients with asthma and bronchitis may lead to thyroid suppression, and if taken by women during pregnancy may produce congenital goitre and hypothyroidism in the newborn. Bromhexine is a synthetic drug which has been shown to increase sputum volume and decrease its viscosity.

Cough suppressants

Cough suppressants, or antitussive agents, are used in the symptomatic treatment of cough. They are of two types:
   1. Drugs which are used primarily to relieve pain, but which also

depress respiration and suppress the cough reflex. Among the more important of these is the opium alkaloid, codeine, and the synthetic compounds pholcodine and dextromethorphan.

2. Drugs which specifically raise the threshold of the cough centre in the brain or which act peripherally to reduce the afferent flow of impulses which stimulate the cough centre. Noscapine, also derived from opium, resembles papaverine in its action on smooth muscle, and has cough suppressant properties while lacking the narcotic effect of morphine and its related compounds. Several of the drugs in this group such as benzonatate, carbetapentane and dimethoxanate have local anaesthetic, atropine-like or antispasmodic properties which probably contribute to their therapeutic effect.

12

Drugs on the gastrointestinal tract

The stomach and intestines have a dual autonomic innervation. The parasympathetic division is responsible for secretion of digestive enzymes, peristalsis and relaxation of sphincters, whereas the sympathetic system produces effects opposite to these. Thus cholinomimetic drugs and anticholinesterases will cause colic and promote defaecation, while anticholinergic drugs relax the bowel and cause constipation. Drugs which block autonomic ganglia reduce both the sympathetic and parasympathetic drive, but constipation ensues as parasympathetic activity is normally predominant. Drugs which selectively block sympathetic nerve terminals, e.g. bethanidine, often cause diarrhoea. Sympathomimetic drugs act on the bowel mainly through α-receptors, but this has little practical significance.

Gastrointestinal secretions can be reduced in volume by anticholinergic drugs, but the treatment of peptic ulcer with these compounds is limited. A more effective approach is the use of an antihistamine which specifically blocks gastric H_2 receptors.

DRUGS IN PEPTIC ULCER

Antacids

Antacids are weak bases which react with hydrochloric acid in the stomach to form a salt. This salt should preferably be non-absorbable, for if it is absorbed, systemic alkalosis can result. This is the major drawback with sodium bicarbonate.

The object of treatment is to produce a prolonged increase in the pH of the stomach, but in practice this is seldom achieved because large quantities (1500 ml) of gastric juice are produced daily, and up to 60 g of sodium bicarbonate per day would be required to reduce usefully its acidity (a pH above 4.0). In addition, antacids often provoke gastric acid production, leading to an 'acid rebound'.

This is particularly marked with calcium salts. All available antacids have too short a duration of action to reduce the acidity of the stomach for long after a single dose. This can be overcome by the use of tablets which are designed to be sucked or chewed and slowly release the antacids which they contain.

Antacids are useful for reducing the pain of uncomplicated peptic ulceration or oesophagitis but they promote healing of ulcers only when given in doses in excess of 1000 μmol daily, quantities which frequently produce diarrhoea. They help little in other forms of indigestion, although the belching promoted by carbon dioxide released from sodium bicarbonate gives relief to some patients. Belching can also be promoted by polymethylsiloxane, an anti-foaming agent.

Sodium bicarbonate. This is rapidly effective in relieving ulcer pain, and is a component of many popular proprietary antacid mixtures. Systemic alkalosis occurs when large doses are taken daily. This leads to execretion of a persistently alkaline urine, which can disturb excretion of other drugs and of calcium. If large quantities of milk or calcium-containing antacid are taken simultaneously, hypercalcaemia and renal calcinosis can occur ('milk-alkali' syndrome). The use of sodium bicarbonate in patients with hypertension, congestive cardiac failure or renal disease is unwise, for the sodium load can be substantial.

Aluminium hydroxide. This has both antacid and adsorbent properties. Aluminium ions cause constipation by an inhibitory action on intestinal smooth muscle. They also inhibit pepsin, although this does not produce any appreciable change in protein digestion. Phosphate ions are bound as insoluble salts, and this can produce hypophosphataemia. Aluminium compounds are sometimes used for this purpose in hyperphosphataemia accompanying renal failure. Tetracycline absorption can be impaired by chelation.

Magnesium salts. Magnesium hydroxide, carbonate and trisilicate are widely used. The first two interact with gastric acid, producing magnesium chloride, which is poorly absorbed but soluble. It acts as an osmotic purgative, as does magnesium sulphate. This is the reason why magnesium antacids are often mixed wth constipating calcium or aluminium antacids. The action of magnesium hydroxide is slower and more prolonged than that of sodium bicarbonate.

Magnesium trisilicate yields magnesium chloride and hydrated silicic acid when it reacts with gastric acid. The silicic acid is gelatinous in consistency and has good absorbent properties, which enhance the antacid effect. Its onset of action, however, is slow. In practice, one of the most satisfactory preparations combining high neutralizing capacity, a rapid but long-lasting effect, absence of rebound hypersecretion, non-absorbability, palatability and safety is a liquid mixture of equal parts of magnesium trisilicate and aluminium hydroxide.

Calcium carbonate. This is an effective antacid and produces a more prolonged reduction in gastric acidity than sodium bicarbonate but rebound hyperacidity can occur. Calcium soaps are formed in the intestine by combination with fatty acids. Frequent use can cause constipation.

H_2-receptor blocking drugs

Histamine is a powerful stimulant of gastric acid secretion but this effect is not blocked by the traditional antihistamines. The development of compounds that antagonize the stomach receptors has lead to the concept of the existence of two receptor subtypes, H_1-receptors mediating the peripheral vascular and bronchial smooth muscle responses to histamine released in allergic reactions and anaphylaxis (p. 232), and H_2-receptors which regulate acid secretion in the stomach. H_2-receptors are also found in the atria and uterus but their role here is uncertain.

It has been suggested that histamine might act as a final common pathway in the secretion of gastric acid, whether it is provoked by gastrin, the synthetic analogue pentagastrin, or by vagus nerve stimulation (e.g. sight or smell of food). This is supported by the observation that cimetidine and ranitidine, which are both H_2-receptor blocking drugs, suppress the acid secretion produced by all of these stimuli. Acid secretion in ulcer patients is likewise reduced, leading not only to symptomatic relief but also healing of the ulcer.

About 75–80% of duodenal and gastric ulcers are endoscopically healed after a 4–6 week course of treatment. However, most patients relapse once again when treatment is stopped, and maintenance treatment on a lower dose may then be necessary. The number of patients requiring surgery has fallen dramatically since the introduction of H_2-receptor blockers. Peptic ulceration caused by the Zollinger-Ellison syndrome also responds, and symptomatic relief occurs in gastro-oesphageal reflux.

Cimetidine was the first H_2-receptor antagonist to be introduced; it is a derivative of the histamine molecule. It has a short elimination half-life of about 2 hours, but suppression of acid secretion can occur for up to 8 hours with a suitable dose. It is excreted largely unchanged in the kidneys and it therefore accumulates in renal disease and in the elderly. It crosses the blood-brain barrier and can cause confusion, drowsiness and disorientation probably by acting on histamine receptors in the central nervous system. An increase in circulating prolactin and gynaecomastia may occur. It inhibits cytochrome P_{450} in hepatic microsomes and thereby reduces drug oxidation; interactions with warfarin, benzodiazepines, phenytoin and propranolol have been reported. Cimetidine also reduces liver blood flow and it is used in upper gastro-intestinal haemorrhage, but this treatment requires further evaluation.

Ranitidine is more potent than cimetidine and a smaller dose is used. It has a similar plasma half-life but only about 70% of the drug is excreted unchanged and therefore it accumulates less in renal disease and in the elderly. Effects on the central nervous system occur less commonly and it does not inhibit microsomal drug metabolism.

Anticholinergic drugs

Anticholinergic drugs can reduce the volume of gastric acid secreted, but have little or no effect on the pH of the empty stomach. After a meal, however, the acidity of the stomach can be decreased by anticholinergics, but the effect is small, for acid production at this time is largely the result of food-stimulated gastrin secretion. In some ulcer patients symptoms may be caused partly by disturbances of gastric motility and muscle spasm, and anticholinergics may help to overcome this.

Unwanted effects are usual in the dosage required to reduce gastric motility, and are the result of peripheral anticholinergic effects. They should not be used in patients with reflux oesophagitis, pyloric stenosis, glaucoma or prostatic hypertrophy.

There is probably little difference between the various anticholinergic drugs, although hyoscine butylbromide, propantheline and poldine have been the most popular for use in peptic ulcer. Pirenzipine is a tricyclic compound which penetrates the blood-brain barrier poorly. It is a potent inhibitor of gastric acid secretion, probably as a result of its anticholinergic properties.

Liquorice derivatives

Extraction of liquorice root yields glycyrrhizinic acid and a variety of residues. These derivatives form the basis of two proprietary preparations. Carbenoxolone sodium is a derivative of glycyrrhizinic acid, and 'Caved-S' contains liquorice residues (deglycyrrhizinized liquorice) as well as several antacids. Both these substances promote healing of gastric ulcers, and when given in positioned-release capsules which burst on passing through the pylorus, healing of duodenal ulcers also occurs. Their therapeutic effect may be due to a number of factors, including an increase in the life span of gastric epithelial cells, an increase in mucus production and a change in its composition, a decrease in hydrogen-ion back-diffusion and an inhibition of peptic activity.

The main difference between these two derivatives lies in their systemic effects. Carbenoxolone has anti-inflammatory properties, partly by stimulation of adrenocortical steroid production. Aldosterone-like effects cause potassium loss, and retention of sodium and chloride. Hypokalaemia can cause lassitude and weakness, and sodium retention can precipitate oedema and heart failure. The drug therefore should not be used in the old and those with heart or renal disease. A sodium-depleting, potassium-retaining diuretic will reverse these effects, but spironolactone also antagonizes the ulcer-healing action. A thiazide diuretic can aggravate hypokalaemia. Plasma potassium should be measured frequently, and potassium supplements given if necessary. Maintenance treatment is impracticable because of the risks of electrolyte imbalance.

Deglycyrrhizinized liquorice does not have these effects, although diarrhoea occasionally occurs.

Other drugs for peptic ulceration

Chelated bismuth. Chelated bismuth salts, e.g. tripotassium dicitratobismuthate, promote healing of gastric and duodenal ulcers, possibly by coating the crater. No important adverse effects have been reported.

Sucralfate. This is a basic aluminium salt of sulphated sucrose which protects the ulcer from the effects of pepsin, acid and possibly bile salts. It is well tolerated, but constipation occasionally occurs.

Drugs affecting gastric emptying

Anticholinergic drugs such as propantheline delay gastric emptying by reducing parasympathetic tone. The absorption of other drugs given concurrently, e.g. paracetamol, can be delayed by this effect. Tricyclic antidepressants, phenothiazines, antihistamines and anti-Parkinsonian drugs are likely to have similar effects as they often have marked anticholinergic actions. On the other hand, metoclopramide promotes gastric emptying and can speed up drug absorption. This effect is taken advantage of during barium meal estimations.

Spasmolytic drugs

Dicyclomine, an anticholinergic drug, is used for infantile pyloric stenosis and evening colic. Other non-anticholinergic drugs with a direct effect on smooth muscle include alverine and mebeverine, which are used as spasmolytics in spastic colon. Peppermint oil is a deflatulant and anti-spasmodic which is also used in this condition.

Enzymes and bile salts

Pancreatin. This is an extract of hog pancreas, and contains amylase, trypsin and lipase. It is used in patients who have steatorrhoea from pancreatic disease, but it is of little value unless protected from gastric acid either by using a preparation with an enteric coating or by giving cimetidine at the same time.

Bile salts. Dehydrocholic acid increases the volume of bile produced by the liver, but not its content of bile salts. It is of limited value and may aggravate pruritus in biliary stasis.

Cholestyramine. This is an anion-exchange resin which removes bile anions in exchange for chloride ions, and can be of value in reducing the pruritus which accompanies biliary cirrhosis and obstructive jaundice. It also lowers the serum cholesterol (bile salts are formed from cholesterol.) and has been shown to reduce the risk of coronary vascular disease in patients with hypercholesterolaemia.

Chenodeoxycholic acid. Cholesterol gall stones occur when bile contains an excess of cholesterol relative to its bile salt and phospholipid content. Chenodeoxycholic acid alters this ratio in favour of bile salts and phospholipids. It dissolves established gall stones and prevents their recurrence. It also reduces plasma triglyceride levels. Chenodeoxycholic acid is metabolised in the liver to lithocholic acid, which is hepatotoxic. It can cause diarrhoea. Ursodeoxycholic acid is a derivative of chenodeoxycholic acid, but is more potent, causes less diarrhoea and is not hepatotoxic.

Cation-exchange resins

These compounds comprise an insoluble polystyrene matrix with an attached, permanently bound anion. The anion attracts cations, but the latter are free to exchange with other cations in the vicinity. In acute renal failure potassium retention occurs, but this can be corrected by an oral Na^+ resin (Resonium A). However, continuous use of this can lead to hypernatraemia, with hypertension and oedema. Calcium resonium overcomes this problem, but even though calcium ions are poorly absorbed hypercalcaemia can occur.

Purgatives

The terms 'purgative', 'laxative', 'aperient' and 'cathartic' should be regarded as synonymous, as attempts at a classification using these terms lead to confusion. 'Purgatives' can be divided into three types according to their mode of action; (a) bulk purgatives, (b) lubricant purgatives, and (c) stimulant purgatives.

Bulk purgatives

These act by increasing the bulk of the intestinal contents, promoting normal peristalsis and defaecation. Three types are available.

(a) Osmotic purgatives, which include salts having a non-absorbable ion, such as magnesium in magnesium sulphate (Epsom salts) or sulphate in sodium sulphate (Glauber's salts) and the polysaccharide, lactulose. They retain water by osmosis, providing liquid bulk.

(b) Hydrophilic colloids, such as methylcellulose, or psyllium which are indigestible plant residues which absorb water, swell, and increase faecal bulk.

(c) Vegetable fibres, such as bran, ispaghula or sterculia, which are also indigestible and provide bulk, but are not colloidal. Large doses have produced intestinal obstruction.

Lubricant purgatives

Liquid paraffin lubricates faecal material in the colon and rectum, and can be useful when straining is undesirable or when defaecation is painful, as in anal fissure or following haemorrhoidectomy, although it can delay healing after anal surgery. It reduces absorption of the fat-soluble vitamins A and D, and can cause paraffinomas in mesenteric lymph nodes with chronic use. It may leak from the anal sphincter. There is a danger of aspiration pneumonia in the elderly.

Dioctyl sodium sulphosuccinate is a substance which lowers surface tension, allowing water to penetrate and soften the faecal matter. It also increases intestinal secretions by stimulating adenyl cyclase.

Glycerine suppositories and soft soap enemata have long been used as local lubricants.

Stimulant purgatives

The drugs included in this group act in a variety of ways, for which the descriptive term 'stimulant' is an oversimplification. Anthracene derivatives, including senna and cascara, are hydrolyzed to trihydroxymethyl anthraquinone (emodin) which stimulates Auerbach's plexus in the bowel wall. They may produce a reddish-brown discolouration of the urine, and are excreted in the milk of lactating mothers. Castor oil is hydrolyzed also, producing ricinoleic acid, which is irritant to the small bowel. Bisacodyl probably acts by stimulating sensory nerve endings in the mucosa of the large bowel. It can be taken orally or given as a suppository. Danthron is similar. Phenolphthalein, stimulates the colonic smooth muscle directly. It is absorbed and re-excreted in bile, and this 'entero-hepatic' circulation prolongs action. Phenolphthalein sensitivity occasionally occurs, leading to a blotchy rash.

Indications and adverse effects

Fortunately the fashion for regular use of purgatives has declined. There is no justification for the use of these drugs in the normal person. Variation in the frequency of defaecation and in the consistency of the faeces is a normal phenomenon, and not an indication for purgation. Usually the administration of a purgative will exaggerate this variation, for complete emptying of the large bowel is usually followed by a period of 2 or 3 days without defaecation. The person who is overconcerned about his bowel habit will see this period as a justification for his regular use of a purgative.

Purgation is indicated in the following situations:

(a) In bowel disease accompanied by chronic constipation e.g. megacolon without aganglionosis.

(b) In the treatment of helmintic infections of the bowel.

(c) Before surgery on the large bowel and rectum. Senna, cascara and bisacodyl, which act on the large bowel, are suitable for this.

(d) Before sigmoidoscopy or radiology of the bowel, although an enema may be more effective.

(e) In local disease of the anus or rectum, such as haemorrhoids or anal fissure. Faecal softeners and bulk purgatives are most suitable.

(f) Following ingestion of poisons.

(g) In constipation produced by drugs, such as opiates and sedatives.

(h) In hepatic encephalopathy.

Most of the irritant purgatives are slow to act, and are given usually last thing at night. Where rapid purgation is required, e.g. after ingestion of poisons, osmotic purgatives are best.

Purgation can produce many adverse effects. Colicky abdominal pain is frequent, and diarrhoea can follow, leading to dehydration and electrolyte imbalance. Chronic purgation can cause diarrhoea, weight loss, hypokalaemia and muscle weakness. Damage to the myenteric plexus of the large bowel can occur. Acute and chronic active hepatitis have been described with purgatives containing oxyphenisatin. Purgatives should never be given to a patient with undiagnosed abdominal pain, for they can precipitate dangerous complications, e.g. burst appendix.

Antidiarrhoeal drugs

Symptomatic treatment for diarrhoea can be given by administering either an adsorbent substance, which adsorbs irritants, or a drug which alters the tone and motility of the bowel. The cause of the diarrhoea should be considered, and specific therapy given at the same time, if indicated. In acute diarrhoea, antibiotics should be administered only if justified on bacteriological grounds. A severe bacterial infection is best treated with systemic antibiotics (e.g. ampicillin) rather than locally-acting non-absorbed compounds (e.g. neomycin).

Charcoal, chalk and kaolin are the most used adsorbents, although pectin is also of value. Kaolin and morphine mixture remains the most popular antidiarrhoeal preparation.

Opiates increase smooth muscle tone in the bowel, and reduce its motility. This property makes them valuable anti-diarrhoeal drugs. Morphine and codeine phosphate are the most used for this purpose, as most of the synthetic or semisynthetic derivatives have less effect on the bowel. One exception is diphenoxylate, a derivative of pethidine, which is contained in a popular proprietary preparation (Lomotil). Loperamide is related to diphenoxylate, but inhibits colonic activity partly by reducing acetylcholine release from parasympathetic terminals in the bowel wall. The dose of morphine required to counteract diarrhoea is small, and systemic effects are rare. Codeine phosphate, however, sometimes produces dizziness and nausea.

Anticholinergic drugs are often included in antidiarrhoeal preparations, although their use is probably irrational, as diarrhoea often results not from excessive peristaltic activity, but from lack of segmental contractions which delay the passage of the bowel contents. A low dose of atropine is included in some preparations (e.g. Lomotil) in order to lessen abuse.

FURTHER READING

Roberts C J C 1983 Treatment in clinical medicine. Gastrointestinal disease. Springer-Verlag, Berlin

13

Drugs on appetite and weight

OBESITY

Medical treatment of obesity depends on the principle that weight loss can only occur when calorie intake falls below calorie expenditure. There is no substitute for this principle, and drugs which are prescribed to produce weight loss or assist dietary management must depend on influencing calorie intake or expenditure.

Increased calorie expenditure

Thyroid hormones in the form of thyroid extract or L-thyroxine are still used by many doctors to increase metabolic rate and produce weight loss. This is undesirable, however, as the doses of these drugs required to produce weight loss may also produce clinical signs of thyroid overactivity and lead to the development of angina pectoris in patients with ischaemic heart disease.

There is evidence that some anorectic drugs, particularly fenfluramine and the biguanides may in addition have peripheral metabolic effects which increase calorie expenditure (see below). The relative importance of appetite-suppressing and calorie-expending actions in producing their weight-reducing effects is uncertain, however.

Reduction of food intake

There have been sporadic attempts to reduce the absorption of food from the intestine by short-circuiting operations which produce a malabsorption state. These are not satisfactory, however, as they may lead to chronic malnutrition and vitamin deficiencies which are not acceptable alternatives to obesity.

(a) Bulk agents

If hunger results from gastric emptiness, then it is reasonable to suppose that ingestion of inert substances which are not absorbed from the gut would relieve hunger without providing calories for weight increase. The most commonly used substance is methylcellulose which is available as tablets or in various food substitutes. Although free from adverse side-effects, its therapeutic value has not been proven satisfactory.

(b) Anorectic drugs

Anorectic drugs suppress appetite, the subjective awareness of hunger. They can be subdivided into three broad categories, those acting primarily on the central nervous system, those acting primarily on peripheral carbohydrate metabolism, and those for which there is evidence for both central and peripheral mechanisms. (Table 13.1).

Table 13.1   Anorectic drugs

1. Centrally acting with stimulant properties	
a) Sympathamimetic amines	amphetamine
	dexamphetamine
	phenmetrazine
	phentermine
	diethylpropion
	phenylpropanolamine
b) Indole derivatives	mazindol
	ciclazindol
2. Drugs influencing peripheral carbohydrate metabolism	
Biguanides	metformin
3. Drugs with central and peripheral actions	
	fenfluramine

1. Centrally acting anorectics. Indirectly acting amines such as amphetamine and its derivatives dexamphetamine, phenmetrazine, diethylpropion, chlorphentamine, phentermine, and phenylpropanolamine, and the indole derivative mazindol, assist patients to adhere to a dietary regime and to lose weight. They are most effective if taken one to one and a half hours before a meal and controlled studies using linear analogue rating scales have demonstrated a significant reduction in appetite by these drugs. Their most important effect is central stimulation, with restlessness, anxiety, insomnia, tolerance and habituation. These are most marked with amphetamine, dexamphetamine and phenmetrazime, resulting in considerable abuse of these compounds with legislation restricting their availability in some countries. There is now general agreement that they should not be prescribed in conditions for which there is alternative treatment without such adverse effects. These stimulant anorectic drugs are thought to act by potentiating central noradrenergic and dopaminergic systems, and it was at one time believed that appetite suppression might be inevitably linked with central stimulation and the risk of dependence. This is now known not to be so, as the trifluoromethyl derivative of amphetamine, fenfluramine, has anorectic and weight reducing properties without producing central stimulation. In fact, it may produce sedation in therapeutic doses. It is probable that the central actions of fenfluramine are mediated through 5HT mechanisms rather than through noradrenergic or dopaminergic pathways.

2. *Drugs primarily influencing peripheral carbohydrate metabolism — the biguanides.* These drugs, of which metformin is the principal member in current use, are alternatives to the sulphonylurea compounds in the oral treatment of diabetes mellitus (page 197). Metformin frequently produces anorexia both in diabetic and non-diabetic patients and for this reason may be the drug of choice in the over-weight maturity onset diabetic patient who is unable to adhere to a diet or in whom diet alone has failed to produce satisfactory weight loss. It is probable, however, that other metabolic effects are mainly responsible for its weight reducing properties, including increased peripheral uptake of glucose and insulin.

3. *Drugs with central and peripheral actions.* There is evidence that the anti-obesity action of fenfluramine involves not only its centrally mediated suppression of appetite (see above) but also peripheral metabolic effects including fat mobilization and increased glucose uptake into skeletal muscle.

Stimulation of appetite

It is sometimes desirable in clinical practice to increase appetite and body weight. Cyproheptadine is an antihistamine and 5HT antagonist which was noticed to increase appetite and weight during an evaluation of its effect on childhood asthma. These properties have been confirmed in controlled clinical trials in underweight patients.

Several other groups of centrally acting drugs including antipsychotic drugs (phenothiazines), antidepressants (tricyclic drugs), benzodiazepine anxiolytics and lithium produce weight increase in some patients when given for psychotherapeutic purposes. Whilst this may be due in part to the clinical improvement associated with their use, it is probable that direct effects on appetite are also involved, although their mechanisms are uncertain.

Further reading

Silverstone T (ed) 1982 Drugs and appetite. Academic Press, London

14

Antidiabetic drugs

INSULIN

Insulin is synthesized in the β-cells of the pancreatic islets and is released in response to hyperglycaemia. It exerts its effect on blood sugar by increasing glucose uptake by peripheral tissues and by reducing the hepatic output of glucose through diminished glyco-genolysis and gluconeogenesis. It also increases protein synthesis, inhibits the mobilization of fatty acids from peripheral fat depots, and promotes the uptake of amino acids and potassium into cells.

Since insulin is a polypeptide it is destroyed in the gut and cannot be given orally. It is completely absorbed after subcutaneous and intramuscular injection, at a rate which depends on the particular preparation used. The half-life of elimination from plasma is between 5 and 10 minutes and is metabolized chiefly in the liver. The duration of action of insulin is therefore dependent on the dose given as well as the absorption characteristics of the particular preparation.

Choice of insulins

Insulins differ in their source and in their absorption character-istics. Insulin can be extracted from beef or pork pancreas and purified by crystallization. Many insulin preparations contain a mixture of insulin from both these sources and the two differ from each other by one terminal amino acid. Both can produce antibody formation in man and although resistance is uncommon, it is generally to the beef component. The crystallized products can be further purified to remove pro-insulin and other precursors of insulin that tend to be more immunogenic than the insulin itself. Such highly purified insulins are less immunogenic and are particu-larly useful for patients who have become resistant to, or have developed local or generalized allergy to conventional insulins, or in children and young adults who are being put on to insulin for the first time. They should also be used for those requiring intermittent insulin therapy, since this mode of use is associated with a higher incidence of allergy and anaphylaxis. Finally, insulin identical to that produced by man can be prepared by modifying porcine insulin or biosynthetically by recombinant DNA techniques. Human insulins are clinically equivalent to the highly purified products, but surprisingly can still sometimes be immunogenic.

Short acting preparations. Insulins can also be classified by their duration of action (see Table 14.1). Soluble insulin generally acts within an hour of administration and has peak effects at 2 to 4 hours, with a duration of action of 6 to 12 hours after subcutaneous administration. It is generally given 15 to 13 minutes before a meal and is chiefly used twice daily in severe insulin-dependent diabetes, particularly in those whose requirements are large and variable. It can be used either alone or in combination with a longer-acting product. It may also be given intravenously for rapid action in emergency or intramuscularly for slightly less rapid action. Soluble insulin has an acid pH which may cause discomfort at the injection site and reduces the rate of drug absorption. Neutral soluble insulin therefore has a more rapid action and is better tolerated.

Table 14.1 Some insulin preparations

	Preparation	Duration of action (hr)
Short acting	Soluble insulin Neutral insulin	6–12
Intermediate acting	Isophane insulin Insulin zinc suspension (amorphous)	18–24 12–16
Long acting	Protamine zinc insulin Insulin zinc suspension (crystalline)	24–36 30–36
Biphasic	Biphasic insulin injection	24

Intermediate preparations. These preparations begin to act between 1 and 3 hours and have a peak effect between 4 and 15 hours. Duration of action is 12 to 24 hours and these agents are used to smooth control in patients already receiving short acting insulins. Isophane insulin is a complex of insulin with protamine and can be mixed with soluble insulin in the same syringe. Insulin zinc suspension is a complex of amorphous insulin with zinc and is also generally used on a twice daily basis.

Long acting insulins. Long acting insulins are produced by complexing insulin with zinc in a crystalline form or by complexing insulin with protamine and zinc to form protamine zinc insulin. The latter can bind short acting insulins and should not be mixed in the same syringe. These agents act within 2 to 8 hours with a peak action between 6 and 30 hours. Their duration of action lies between 24 and 36 hours. They are generally given once daily to patients with a lesser degree of insulin deficiency, particularly elderly subjects.

Biphasic insulins. These are generally a fixed mixture of short acting and intermediate acting insulins, usually soluble and isophane in fixed proportions (generally 50/50 or 30/70 soluble to isophane). Although convenient for those subjects who find difficulty in mixing insulins themselves, they provide less flexibility in control.

Indications for use of insulin

Three quarters of diabetics do not require insulin therapy. These are generally those with non-insulin-dependent (Type II, or maturity onset) diabetes and have only a relative deficiency of insulin secretion. They may also have abnormal secretory patterns of insulin production and diminished peripheral insulin responsiveness. Most patients not requiring insulin are over 40 years of age and there is often a strong family history of non-insulin-dependent diabetes. Insulin is generally used in the other group of diabetics, those with insulin-dependent (Type I, or juvenile onset) diabetes. Such patients often have an absolute deficiency of insulin synthesis and/or secretion because of β-cell dysfunction. They include all diabetic children, most diabetics under 40 years, but also a few diabetics older than 40 years. Such patients may present with severe complications of diabetes. Insulin may also be needed in those with Type II diabetes which has not responded adequately to dietary control and oral hypoglycaemic drugs, or in patients who, although formerly stable on diet or oral drugs, become unstable because of intercurrent disease. It is impossible to maintain normoglycaemia in the majority of diabetics, even if the insulin is given frequently, but there is evidence that the tightest possible control of plasma glucose will protect from some of the complications of diabetes. Good control is best achieved by monitoring blood glucose and subsequent adjustment of the dose and frequency of insulin administration. Control should be particularly rigid in diabetic pregnancy, in which insulin requirements increase variably.

Diabetic emergencies

Ketoacidosis. In this diabetic emergency the immediate priority is rehydration with normal saline since patients may be markedly dehydrated (average deficit 5L). Potassium supplements are also necessary together with sodium bicarbonate if the arterial pH is less than 7.1. Soluble insulin should be given, ideally as a slow intravenous infusion at a rate of approximately 5 units per hour for an adult, until the plasma glucose concentration has fallen to 10 mm/l. Alternatively, the soluble insulin can be given intramuscularly as an initial loading dose of 20 units followed by 6 units given each hour until the same plasma glucose concentration is reached. Absorption from the intramuscular site may be impaired and erratic if the patient is hypotensive, or has poor peripheral perfusion.

Hyperosmolar coma. In this rarer diabetic emergency, the patient has a relative deficit of water compared with saline and has hypernatraemia and marked hyperglycaemia. Treatment is as for diabetic ketoacidosis, except that half normal saline may be necessary and intravenous heparin should be used to reduce the risks of thrombosis seen with this complication.

Lactic acidosis. This rare complication is more likely in diabetics on biguanides, although its incidence is lower with metformin than it was with the now withdrawn agent, phenformin. The patient is generally only mildly ketotic, but has marked metabolic acidosis due to an accumulation of lactic acid in the blood. Insulin is given, as in other causes of hyperglycaemia, but large amounts of intravenous bicarbonate are necessary and dialysis may be required in very severe cases if the amounts of sodium bicarbonate which are needed lead to sodium overdose. Mortality in this condition is high.

Hypoglycaemic coma. This is the most commonest adverse effect of insulin and is associated with sweating, tachycardia and palpitations, mental confusion and eventually coma and convulsions if left untreated. Treatment is with oral glucose or sucrose, or if necessary (up to 50 ml of 50% solution for intravenous infusion). If it is impossible to give the glucose intravenously, glucagon (1 mg) can be given intramuscularly or subcutaneously, repeated if necessary after 10 minutes. This corrects hypoglycaemia by promoting hepatic glycogenolysis and may not be effective in situations where hepatic glycogen is already deplated. After the patient has responded, glucose should be given orally to prevent a recurrence of hypoglycaemia.

ORAL HYPOGLYCAEMIC DRUGS

Sulphonylureas

These are structurally related to sulphonamides and reduced blood sugar primarily by increasing insulin secretion. Some functioning islet cells in the pancreas are necessary for these agents to be effective and they are therefore used most often in patients with non-insulin-dependent diabetes mellitus. They also inhibit gluconeogenesis and insulin degradation in the liver and may increase the number of insulin receptors peripherally. Tolbutamide and glibenclamide have a similar half-life (5–8 hours) and therefore similar duration of action of around 6 to 10 hours. They are metabolized by the liver to inactive metabolites. Tolbutamide is generally given twice daily, but glibenclamide can be given as a once or twice daily dose. Chlorpropramide is partly metabolized, but mostly excreted unchanged in the urine. The half-life is around 36 hours although the duration of action can be as long as 60 hours. It is generally given as a single dose. Glymidine is structurally different from the sulphonylureas. It has a half-life of between 3 and 6 hours and a duration of action similar to tolbutamide and glibenclamide, and can be given once or twice daily. It may be tried with care in patients who have sulphonylurea hypersensitivity.

Adverse effects. Adverse effects are uncommon and include gastrointestinal intolerance with nausea, vomiting, diarrhoea and anorexia. Hypersensitivity is much rarer, but may present with skin rash and jaundice, or blood dyscrasias. Alcohol intolerance, characterized by facial flushing, may occur after chlorpropamide and tolbutamide, but is uncommon after glibenclamide. Hypoglycaemia is an important adverse effect, particularly with the longer acting chlorpropramide. It is more common in patients with diminished renal function, e.g. the elderly. A shorter acting agent which is metabolized by the liver is therefore preferable in elderly patients.

Biguanides

Metformin is now the only available biguanide because its predecessor, phenformin, was associated with a unacceptably high incidence of lactic acidosis. Unlike the sulphonylureas, it does not promote insulin release from the pancreas, but promotes peripheral uptake of both glucose and insulin. Metformin is therefore only of value in patients who have some insulin production. Metformin is excreted unchanged by the kidney with a half-life of approximately 2 hours, and it must therefore be given at 8 to 12 hour intervals.

Adverse effects. The major adverse side effects are anorexia, nausea, vomiting and diarrhoea. Although the anorectic effect may contribute to weight loss and subsequent improvement in diabetic control it can be so severe that the patient is unable to tolerate metformin. Lactic acidosis remains a rare but potentially very serious adverse effect. It is more common in patients with impaired renal or hepatic function, in alcoholism or in those with intercurrent illnesses.

Indications for use of oral hypoglycaemics

Dietary control of non-insulin dependent diabetes is the most important single measure which will be sufficient to control a third of patients. Sulphonylureas tend to encourage weight gain and are therefore used in patients whose diabetes has not been adequately controlled after reduction in body weight to within 15% of the ideal. Biguanides are preferable to sulphonylureas in markedly obese patients and if one type of oral hypoglycaemic drug is ineffective, a combination of sulphonylures and biguanide may be useful. Even if the patient is adequately controlled by oral hypoglycaemic agents, these should be replaced by insulin during pregnancy, surgery, intercurrent infection or ketosis.

15

Drugs in endocrinology

THE HYPOTHALAMUS AND PITUITARY

The pituitary is responsible for the secretion of a number of important hormones, but is dependent upon the integrity of the hypothalamus to carry out this function. The posterior pituitary develops embryologically as an outgrowth from the brain, and remains connected to the hypothalamus by two important tracts of nerve fibres which act as channels down which the two posterior pituitary hormones are transported. The supraoptic nucleus situated above the optic chiasma in the hypothalamus produces vasopressin (antidiuretic hormone, ADH) which is transported down the supraoptico-hypophyseal tract to the pituitary, where it is released as needed from the nerve terminals. Oxytocin is produced in the paraventricular nucleus and is released from the pituitary in the same way. The connections are illustrated in Fig. 15.1.

The anterior pituitary is derived from the foregut, not the brain, and is not connected to the hypothalamus by nervous pathways. Instead, a portal circulation develops which carries venous blood containing polypeptide hormones known as 'releasing factors' from the hypothalamus to a second capillary bed in the anterior pituitary. These factors liberate the anterior pituitary hormones from their granular stores. Releasing hormones have been described for thyroid-stimulating hormone (TSH), the gonadotrophins (follicle-stimulating hormone, FSH, and luteinizing hormone, LH), prolactin, adrenocorticotrophin (ACTH) and melanocyte-stimulating hormone (MSH). The structures of two of releasing hormones, thyrotrophin-releasing hormone (TRH) and gonadotrophin-releasing hormone (LH/FSH-RH), are known.

The release of two hormones, prolactin and growth hormone (GH), and possibly a third, MSH, are also controlled by release-inhibiting hormones. The structure of growth hormone release-inhibiting hormone is known. Dopamine may be the prolactin

199

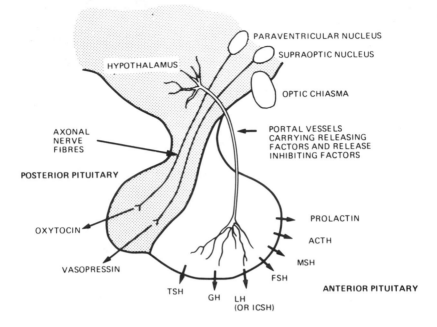

Fig. 15.1 Mechanisms controlling the secretion of pituitary hormones.

release-inhibiting factor. Drugs which impair dopaminergic transmission, such as phenothiazines, reserpine, α-methyldopa and metoclopramide, can cause hyperprolactinaemia and galactorrhoea by impairing the inhibitory control of prolactin release.

POSTERIOR PITUITARY HORMONES

Vasopressin (ADH)

In physiological amounts vasopressin acts on the distal and collecting tubules of the kidney, increasing their permeability to water and thereby conserving water. The absence of this hormone produces diabetes insipidus. This occurs as a permanent feature only when the supraoptic region of the hypothalamus is destroyed. Posterior pituitary damage causes only temporary derangement of vasopressin secretion. In larger doses the hormone produces a pressor response by peripheral vasoconstriction, angina from coronary vasoconstriction, and abdominal colic.

For clinical use vasopressin is available as pitressin of pig or beef origin, or in the synthetic forms of lysine-vasopressin (LVP) or desmopressin. Pitressin of animal origin is usually administered as pitressin tannate in oil, which acts for a longer time than aqueous solutions and is suitable for long term management of diabetes insipidus. It needs to be given intramuscularly every 1 to 3 days. Repeated injection into the same area of skin can lead to accumulation of oil and impaired absorption of the hormone. Pitressin powder in the form of a snuff is available but should no longer be used as it can produce allergic reactions in the nose and lungs, and chronic use can lead to atrophic rhinitis from the vasoconstrictor effect of the preparation. Poor absorption results. The aqueous preparation is used in conjunction with water deprivation as a diagnostic test for diabetes insipidus.

Some of the above disadvantages have been overcome by the introduction of synthetic lysine vasopressin. This is administered by nasal spray, which is more convenient than injection for the patient, but it can produce nasal congestion and ulceration of the mucosa. It has a short duration of action, having to be repeated up to six times daily, and it may be inadequate alone in severe diabetes insipidus.

Another synthetic analogue, desmopressin (1-desamino-8-D-arginine vasopressin, DDAVP), is as potent as lysine vasopressin but has a more prolonged action, allowing satisfactory control with twice-daily administration of an intranasal spray. It has no pressor activity and no smooth muscle contracting properties.

Aqueous vasopressin has found a further use in the treatment of bleeding oesophageal varices. It lowers the portal blood pressure by producing splanchnic vasoconstriction, and thus the bleeding from anastomotic vessels is reduced. It also promotes the passage of blood clot through the intestine, reducing the likelihood of hepatic coma from digestion of blood proteins.

Treatment of diabetes insipidus. Although vasopressin is the mainstay of treatment, oral agents have been sought because of their convenience. Sulphonylureas, particularly chlorpropamide, reduce polyuria in hypothalamic diabetes insipidus, but not in the nephrogenic form of the disease, which is caused by renal insensitivity to the circulating hormone. They sensitize the renal tubules to diminished amounts of circulating vasopressin, but are ineffective when there is a complete absence of the hormone, e.g. post-hypophysectomy. Chlorpropamide requires about 3 days to produce its effect. It can control mild diabetes insipidus when given alone, but in more severe disease the addition of vasopressin is necessary. Dilutional hyponatraemia can occur if the level of circulating vasopressin is fluctuating, or if chlorpropamide and vasopressin are given together without water restriction. Hypoglycaemia may also occur. Thiazide diuretics are less effective than chlorpropamide in hypothalamic diabetes insipidus, but unlike the latter drug they have a clinically useful effect in the nephrogenic type, especially if sodium intake is restricted at the same time. Oral potassium supplements are necessary to avoid hypokalaemia.

Oxytocin

Oxytocin causes a contraction of uterine smooth muscle, the sensitivity of which gradually increases during pregnancy. Although the role of this hormone during normal labour is not clear, when given by intravenous infusion it induces labour, and is widely used for this purpose. Dangerously powerful contractions can be produced by excessive doses. Oxytocin is released by stimulation of afferent fibres of the lactating breast, and it causes contraction of the myoepithelial cells with ejection of milk. This accounts for the uterine contractions which accompany breast-feeding postpartum. Oxytocin is usually given in a synthetic form, although an extract of mammalian pituitary glands is still available.

Other drugs acting on the uterus

Ergometrine. It is now standard procedure in obstetric practice to administer intramuscular ergometrine on the crowning of the fetal head. By the time the placenta has been delivered the drug is producing its effect. Ergometrine has a direct stimulant action on the uterine muscle, causing a rapid contraction of the uterus and a reduced incidence of postpartum haemorrhage. Ergotamine also stimulates the uterus, but its more powerful peripheral vasoconstrictor action makes it less suitable for obstetric use. In addition to their direct effects on smooth muscle both drugs have an α-adrenolytic activity, but this is of no therapeutic value. A preparation (Syntometrine) combining synthetic oxytocin and ergometrine is available, and produces more rapid contraction of the uterus than ergometrine alone.

Prostaglandins. Amongst their many actions prostaglandins of the E and F series stimulate the myometrium. Their presence in human seminal, menstrual and amniotic fluids, and in the maternal circulation during labour and abortion, suggests that they may have an important role in uterine function during conception and labour. Prostaglandins E_2 and $F_{2\alpha}$ are widely used both orally and by intravenous infusion for induction of labour and abortion, and are given to promote cervical ripening. Prostaglandin $F_{2\alpha}$ produces more side-effects, notably nausea, vomiting and diarrhoea.

Non-steroidal anti-inflammatory drugs. By inhibiting prostaglandin synthesis, aspirin and other anti-inflammatory drugs inhibit uterine motility and have therefore been used to inhibit preterm labour. Unfortunately, they can cross the placental barrier and can cause premature closure of the ductus arteriosus, leading to primary pulmonary hypertension of the newborn. They are therefore contraindicated in pregnancy and labour. Non-steroidal anti-inflammatory drugs are being used in patent-ductus arteriosus in neonates (p. 159).

Sympathomimetic drugs. Stimulation of β-adrenergic receptors in the uterus produces relaxation of the myometrium. Isoxsuprine, ritodrine, orciprenaline and salbutamol, all having predominant β²-mimetic activity, are of value in arresting premature labour.

ANTERIOR PITUITARY HORMONES

Growth hormone

Growth hormone has several functions, (a) it promotes longitudinal growth of long bones, (b) it is concerned in the growth and maturation of the viscera and soft tissues, (c) it elevates the blood glucose level by anti-insulin action, and (d) it stimulates protein synthesis and fat breakdown. Its effects on bone growth are dependent upon the levels of circulating sex hormones, for the latter are responsible for bone maturation and fusion of the epiphyses, and growth hormone can only produce lengthening when the epiphyses are unfused. Thus an excess of growth hormone with normal levels of sex hormones during childhood produces gigantism, whereas in adults it will lead to the clinical features of acromegaly. A deficiency of growth hormone in childhood produces patients of short stature and with delayed puberty, although they eventually become fertile. It is important to institute replacement therapy at the earliest opportunity in these children.

Growth hormone is a polypeptide comprising 188 amino acids. It has not been synthesized, and because of species differences in structure, growth hormone obtained from any source other than man or monkey is of no value in treating patients. In the United Kingdom human growth hormone was extracted from pituitary glands collected at post-mortem by pathologists throughout the country, and distributed by the Medical Research Council. Human growth hormone produced by recombinant DNA techniques has been manufactured to take the place of this material because of concern about transmission of neurotropic viruses. Replacement therapy is effective in stimulating growth in children whose small stature is due to growth hormone deficiency, but in other types of dwarfism response is disappointing.

Growth-hormone release-inhibiting hormone (GH-RIH, somatostatin), whose structure has been characterized, regulates the pituitary release of growth hormone. Development of a long-acting preparation should prove a major advance in the treatment of acromegaly. It also reduces insulin and glucagon secretion by a direct action on the pancreas, which may be of future therapeutic value.

The semi-synthetic ergot alkaloid, bromocriptine (α-bromo ergocriptine) reduces elevated growth hormone levels and relieves the symptoms of acromegaly. It has been an important advance in the management of this condition. It stimulates dopamine receptors in the CNS.

Prolactin

Raised levels of circulating prolactin have been demonstrated in patients with galactorrhoea from a variety of causes, among which are a number of drugs, including phenothiazines, metoclopramide, reserpine, imipramine, haloperidol, α-methyldopa and oral contraceptives. All but the last of these impair dopaminergic transmission, which account for their ability to produce this effect. As the secretion of prolactin from the pituitary is held in check by a hypothalamic inhibitory factor, probably dopamine, galactorrhoea is the result of a suppression of the release of this factor or by blockade of its effects on the pituitary.

The dopamine agonist drug, bromocriptine, reduces raised serum prolactin levels and is used in treating galactorrhoea associated with amenorrhea. Galactorrhoea responds rapidly and normal menstrual periods are restored within a few weeks. Bromocriptine can be used in the presence of a pituitary tumour. In amenorrhoeic patients with a normal prolactin level, no response is seen. Its dopamine agonist properties probably explain its therapeutic effect.

Gonadotrophins

Antibodies are quickly developed to gonadotrophins of animal origin so human material has to be used in treating gonadotrophin deficiency. Although they can be extracted from pituitary glands, human menopausal urinary gonadrotrophin (HMG) is rich in FSH and LH and this is the usual source of these hormones. Human chorionic gonadotrophin (HCG), obtained from the urine of pregnant women, has actions similar to those of LH and is often used in conjunction with HMG.

Gonadotrophin deficiency causes delayed puberty in children, impotence and infertility in adult males, and oligo- or amenorrhoea with infertility in women. In order to promote ovulation in women HMG is given until an ovarian response has been detected, as judged by clinical signs of oestrogenic effects and by increasing levels of urinary oestrogen, and then HCG is given to induce ovulation. Infertility from causes other than gonadotrophin deficiency does not respond to this treatment. In males HCG has the same effect as ICSH (LH) and can be used to stimulate testosterone production from the interstitial cells, which leads to the development of secondary sexual characteristics in patients with delayed puberty. Spermatogenesis is stimulated by HMG, but prolonged treatment is required, sometimes with ICSH supplements.

Clomiphene. Clomiphene is a gonadotrophin-releasing agent, acting by blocking the negative feedback receptor sites in the hypothalamus. It is used in the diagnosis and treatment of hypogonadism and infertility. In patients who have low circulating levels of gonadotrophins a failure to increase these levels after administration of clomiphene suggests a hypothalamic-pituitary cause. Treatment with clomiphene can often induce ovulation in infertile hypo- or normogonadotrophic women.

Thyroid stimulating hormone

TSH stimulates the uptake of iodine by the thyroid gland and promotes release of thyroxine and triiodothyronine. It is used diagnostically in hypothyroidism to distinguish intrinsic thyroid disease from a disorder of hypothalamic-pituitary function. When the thyroid gland is normal, TSH will cause a release of thyroid hormones. It is also of value for assessing thyroid function in patients already receiving thyroxine, or in identifying metastases from a thyroid carcinoma, for it promotes uptake of radio-iodine, which can be assessed by scanning. TSH is of bovine origin, and allergic reactions to it can occur.

Thyrotrophin-releasing hormone (TRH), whose structure has been elucidated, can be used diagnostically to distinguish between primary hypothyroidism and that secondary to pituitary disease.

Adrenocorticotrophic hormone (see page 231)

THYROID HORMONES

The thyroid gland secretes a mixture of thyroxine (T_4) and triiodo-thyronine (T_3) in the ratio of 50:1. They are synthesized in the thyroid gland by iodination of tyrosine, forming mono- and di-iodotyrosine, which subsequently conjugate to form T_3 and T_4 (Fig. 15.2). All these reactions occur while the constituents are bound to thyroglobulin, and the hormones have to be split off by a protease enzyme before they can enter the circulation. T_3 is about four times more potent than T_4 in increasing the metabolic rate, and thus both hormones contribute to the metabolic effects produced by thyroid secretions. In hyperthyroidism there is usually an increase in both hormones, but occasionally only the T_3 fraction is elevated.

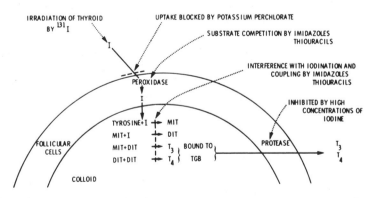

Fig. 15.2 Synthesis of thyroid hormones and its modification by antithyroid drugs.

Treatment of hypothyroidism

T_4 is usually used for replacement therapy. There is seldom an indication for giving T_3. Thyroid extract, prepared from pork or beef thyroid glands, contains both hormones, but this preparation is poorly standardized and therefore variable in its effects. As T_4 can be synthesized and precisely standardized, it has rendered thyroid extract obsolete.

Synthetic T_4 is the sodium salt of L-thyroxine. For full replacement 200 to 300 μg daily are required. One to two weeks is required for its effects to become maximal, and they persist for several weeks after discontinuing treatment. The reason for this is that T_4 is about 99.9% protein bound in serum and tissues, so it takes some days to saturate these physiologically-inactive stores. Caution should be exercised in administering the drug to the elderly or those with ischaemic heart disease, in whom angina of effort or heart failure can be precipitated. The dose should be increased cautiously, and rarely needs to be greater than 200 μg daily. Addition of a β-adrenergic blocker may reduce the occurrence of angina. Monitoring the serum TSH level will assist in tailoring the dosage to suit the patient; the level will fall to normal when the optimum dose has been achieved.

Liothyronine is the sodium salt of triiodothyronine. Being less protein bound it acts more quickly than T_4, the peak effect occurring about 48 hours after a single dose. There are two indications for its use in preference to T_4, (a) in the treatment of myxoedema coma, and (b) when it is necessary to stop treatment from time to time to perform scanning studies, e.g. in looking for secondaries after surgical treatment of a thyroid carcinoma.

For the treatment of myxoedema coma it is usual to give 10 to 20 μg of T_3 and 50 mg of hydrocortisone hemisuccinate intravenously every 12 hours initially, but oral administration of T_4 should begin as soon as possible. Administration of hydrocortisone is of utmost importance as prolonged hypothyroidism usually depresses adrenocortical function, and the increase in metabolic activity produced by T_3 puts immediate demands on this.

Treatment of hyperthyroidism

The object of treatment is to reduce the synthesis and release of thyroid hormones. This can be done in several ways, as are summarized in Fig. 15.2.

Potassium perchlorate. Uptake of iodine is blocked by this drug, but the block can be overcome by a modest intake of iodine, e.g. in a cough mixture. Agranulocytosis and fatal aplastic anaemia occur rarely, but with sufficient frequency for its use to be reserved for those patients who cannot tolerate an imidazole or thiouracil derivative.

Imidazoles. Carbimazole is the drug of first choice. It inhibits, by substrate competition, the peroxidase enzyme which releases iodine from circulating iodides, and, in addition, it inhibits the enzymes responsible for iodination of tyrosine and coupling of the iodinated derivatives. There is some evidence that carbimazole may also have an immunosuppressant effect in Graves' disease. It is suitable for use in most types of hyperthyroidism where drug therapy is preferred to surgery or radio-iodine treatment. The starting dose is chosen according to the severity of the disease. The object is to render the patient euthyroid and then to reduce to a maintenance dose. Concurrent administration of T_4 prevents hypothyroidism and avoids difficulty in dose titration. Withdrawal of the drug is often possible after one to two years, although relapse occurs in a proportion of patients.

Methimazole is similar.

Hypothyroidism and enlargement of the thyroid can occur with excessive doses of an imidazole. Rashes occur often, and agranulocytosis is seen occasionally.

Thiouracils. Propyl- and methylthiouracil have actions resembling those of the imidazoles. They are usually reserved for those patients who are intolerant of the latter drugs.

Iodine and iodides. In pharmacological doses iodine or potassium iodide cause inhibition of the release of T_3 and T_4 from the colloidal stores of the thyroid gland. Their use is reserved for the preoperative preparation of patients for thyroidectomy, because the vascularity of the gland is reduced by these compounds. The effect is transient and therefore the operation should be performed 2 to 3 weeks after starting treatment. In other than mild cases previous treatment with a thiouracil or imidazole is necessary. Iodine should not be given immediately after treatment with potassium perchlorate, for it can produce a thyroid crisis by sudden release of hormones. Iodine or iodine-containing medicines (e.g. cough mixtures) taken during pregnancy can cause a goitre in the fetus.

Radioactive iodine. Because iodine is concentrated in the thyroid gland, a small dose of radioactive iodine will irradiate the hormone-producing follicular cells. [131]I has been widely used for this purpose, and is a valuable alternative to surgery. It should not be used in children or in women of childbearing age. One of the chief disadvantages of this treatment is the frequency with which post-irradiation hypothyroidism occurs. For this reason ^{125}I is undergoing trials. In theory this isotope might be preferable because its emission is less penetrating than that of ^{131}I, and should cause less damage of the nuclei of the follicular cells, but assessment of its possible advantages must await the results of long-term follow-up in these trials.

Adrenergic-blocking drugs. β-receptor blocking drugs can reduce the heart rate and peripheral manifestations of hyperthyroidism, and can therefore be useful as an adjunct to treatment with anti-thyroid drugs. Blocking drugs without intrinsic sympathomimetic properties, such as propranolol, are preferable. Heart failure is not an absolute contraindication to propranolol so long as vigorous treatment with digoxin and diuretics is started simultaneously.

Treatment of exophthalmos

In some patients with hyperthyroidism, exophthalmos is troubling or even threatening to the eyes. Unfortunately, it usually does not respond to treatment of the hyperthyroid state, although the accompanying lid retraction is reduced. The levator palpebrae is partly composed of adrenergically innervated smooth muscle, and the adrenergic nerve blocking drug guanethidine usually relieves lid retraction when instilled into the lacrynmal sac. Unfortunately, it often aggravates the grittiness of the conjunctiva which occurs in the exophthalmic eye. Methylcellulose drops can help by lubricating the conjunctiva and lids. In severe cases corticosteroids or surgical decompression of the orbit is necessary.

Parathyroid hormone and calcitonin

The principle physiological function of parathyroid hormone is to maintain a normal plasma calcium level. It does so probably by effects on bone metabolism, and on the renal excretion and intestinal absorption or calcium. These effects are closely interrelated with the tissue effects of vitamin D. A parenteral preparation containing parathyroid extract is available and is used diagnostically as well as in the treatment of tetany. It is too antigenic for long-term use in hypoparathyroidism, the management of which depends upon administration of vitamin D or dihydrotachysterol (see p. 242).

The normal physiological role of calcitonin is uncertain, but it is capable of reducing elevated calcium levels. Preparations are available containing either porcine or synthetic salmon calcitonin. The latter is less antigenic and is proving useful in inhibiting the excessive bone resorption and relieving bone pain in Paget's disease, and in the management of severe hypercalcaemia.

SEX HORMONES

Androgens and anabolic steroids

Androgens have two main types of action, (a) development of the secondary sexual characteristics of the male and growth of the genitalia, and (b) anabolic effects, such as retention of nitrogen, synthesis of body proteins, development of the musculature and bones, and fusion of the epiphyses. It has been possible to separate partly these effects so that some compounds have predominant anabolic actions, and although they are widely used in patients with chronic debilitating diseases the evidence that they promote recovery is conflicting.

Androgenic preparations

Testosterone is the chief androgen secreted by the testes and adrenal cortex under the pituitary control of ICSH. Testosterone is converted to its active metabolite, 5-α-dihydrotestosterone, in the target cells. A deficiency of this hormone starting in childhood produces eunuchoidism, but when it starts after puberty it causes a regression of secondary sexual characteristics, loss of libido and infertility. Testosterone is used for replacement therapy, but the unmodified molecule is rapidly metabolized. Esterification lengthens the duration of action. It can be given in a number of ways, sublingually as testosterone propionate in a waxy base, intramuscularly as the propionate in water or oenanthate in oil, or by subcutaneous implantation as testosterone pellets. Flumesterone, a synthetic androgen, can be given orally. Methyltestosterone is available for sublingual administration, but it is poorly absorbed and occasionally causes cholestatic jaundice.

Indication for use of androgens

(a) *Replacement therapy in hypogonadism.* Testosterone will induce sexual development when puberty is delayed, and will restore potency and libido in adults who have developed androgen deficiency, regardless of whether it is due to testicular or pituitary disorder. When the deficiency is secondary to pituitary disease, however, it is preferable to use HCG to induce puberty. Fertility can be restored only if the seminiferous tubules of the testes are functional, and are stimulated by administration of gonadotrophins.

(b) *Growth disorders*. Growth can be curtailed by stimulating epiphyseal fusion in boys growing to an excessive height. Although an initial growth spurt is produced in dwarfism, early fusion of the epiphyses can cause greater curtailment of growth than would have occurred in the absence of treatment, especially if used in excessive dosage.

Anabolic steroids

A number of these are available, the more important being nandrolone, methanolone, methandienone and norethandrolone. These compounds are used to encourage protein anabolism in chronic disease, following major surgery or in patients with 'senile' osteoporosis, but there is no good evidence as yet that they are of real value. Their ability to reduce protein catabolism is used to delay uraemia in patients with acute renal failure. Androgens or anabolic steroids are sometimes of value in inhibiting the growth of a breast carcinoma, particularly in premenopausal women, and in the management of aplastic anaemia. Oxymethalone is the drug of choice in the latter. Although anabolic steroids have less marked androgenic properties than testosterone, they can cause masculinization in women. They will also cause masculinization of the fetus if used during pregnancy.

Oestrogens

Oestrogens are produced mainly in the ovary and placenta, but small amounts are synthesized in the adrenal and testes. The three important oestrogens are oestrone, oestradiol and oestriol. The last of these is a physiologically active metabolite of oestradiol, and is produced in large quantities by the placenta. Its main effects are on the cervix and vaginal epithelium, while oestradiol influences endometrial development.

For therapeutic use oestrogens can be given in a variety of forms, but essentially these can be divided into two classes, (a) naturally occurring steroid hormones or their derivatives, and (b) synthetic non-steroid compounds with oestrogenic effects.

Steroid hormones and derivatives. Naturally-occurring hormones have a rather short-lived effect because they are metabolized quickly. A number of derivatives of oestradiol have been produced and these form the basis of many preparations. Two orally-active derivatives, ethinyloestradiol and mestranol, are widely used, and most combined oestrogen-progestogen contraceptive pills are based on these two oestrogens. Oestradiol monobenzoate is a longer acting parenteral preparation which is slowly hydrolyzed to release oestradiol. Oestradiol valerate can be injected as an oily solution from which it is slowly absorbed.

One proprietary preparation, Premarin, contains natural oestrogens, equilin and equilenin, which are extracted from mare's urine.

Non-steroid oestrogens. Stilboestrol is the most important of these and is active orally. Alternative drugs are dienoestrol, methallenoestril, and chlorotrianisene.

Indications for oestrogen therapy

(a) Menorrhagia can be controlled by administration of oestrogens in high dosage, but a gradual tailing-off is necessary if withdrawal bleeding is not to be precipitated. This problem, however, has been largely overcome by the use of oestrogen-progestogen combinations, for the progestogen produces secretory changes in the endometrum which prevent severe bleeding. High doses of oestrogens can cause nausea.

(b) Climacteric symptoms respond to oestrogen treatment, but often at the expense of some degree of post menopausal bleeding. Oestriol produces little or no bleeding. Oestrogens prevent excess bone loss following premature menopause.

(c) Amenorrhoea is usually caused by hypothalamic-pituitary disorder rather than ovarian disease, and oestrogen-withdrawal bleeding can usually be induced. Accompanying underdevelopment of secondary sexual characteristics will respond to oestrogen administration, but infertility will not. Gonadotrophin or clomiphene treatment is necessary to induce ovulation. Oligomenorrhoea may be worsened by oestrogen treatment, which can further disrupt the pituitary-ovarian feedback mechanism.

(d) Endometriosis can often be cured by prolonged use of oestrogen-progestogen combinations, but the use of progesterone preparations alone is found satisfactory by some. The aim is to produce atrophy of the ectopic endometrial tissue.

(e) The use of stilboestrol in the treatment of threatened abortion has been discontinued since it was recognised that vaginal adenocarcinoma could occur in the adolescent daughters of mothers treated with the drug.

(f) Lactation can be suppressed in mothers who do not wish to breast feed. Bromocriptine is preferable to oestrogens for this purpose, however, because it specifically reduces prolactin levels by acting on the pituitary. However, in practice simpler methods usually suffice e.g. avoiding nipple stimulation and breast support.

(g) Carcinoma of the prostate often responds dramatically to oestrogen therapy, but feminization and thrombo-embolic disease can be produced.

Progestogens

Progesterone is produced naturally by the corpus luteum and placenta, and it has two main functions, (a) to induce secretory changes in the endometrium in the luteal phase of the menstrual cycle, and (b) to maintain pregnancy after implantation of the ovum. Progestogens are used therapeutically to encourage these effects when natural control seems to be lacking.

Progesterone itself is very insoluble and has a short half-life in the body. Although it can be given in oil, synthetic substitutes are preferable. These are derived from two steroid substances, nortestosterone and 17α-hydroxyprogesterone. Nortestosterone is derived from testosterone by demethylation, and from it are produced the most-used synthetic progestogens, norethisterone, norethynodrel, lynestrenol and ethynodiol. These compounds have marked progestogenic effects, but, with the exception of allylestrenol, they retain slight androgenic properties which make them unsuitable for use during early pregnancy, because they can have a virilizing effect in the fetus. In the adult female, however, these effects are negligible. They are metabolized to a small extent to oestrogenic substances, which give them oestrogenic properties in addition. However, they are usually administered in combination with oestrogens in order to suppress ovulation for contraceptive purposes and for the treatment of menstrual disorders.

17α-Hydroxyprogesterone is an intermediate in the biosynthesis of cortisol, but is not secreted as a progestogen by the adrenal cortex. Esterification of this compound yields megestrol acetate, which has a negligible oestrogenic or androgenic effect, and is suitable for use in pregnant women.

Indications for progestogen therapy

Menstrual disorders. A combination of oestrogen and progestogen will impose a regular menstrual pattern in most cases of menorrhagia and metrorrhagia. Dysmenorrhoea often disappears, and endometriosis can be cured by long-term use of these combinations. Symptoms of premenstrual tension often respond to non-oestrogenic progestogens given alone. Bromocriptine is known to reduce breast discomfort, but its role in treatment is uncertain.

To prevent abortion. Progestogens are still widely used for preventing threatened abortion or premature labour, although it is likely that they are of value only when there is a deficiency of maternal progestogens. Allylestrenol is to be preferred because it is non-virilizing.

Carcinoma of the uterine body. Progestogens are useful in treating metastases after the primary has been excised.

The contraceptive pill

The pills most widely used are combinations of a progestogen and an oestrogen (see Table 15.1). Only two oestrogenic compounds are used in the pill whereas a variety of progestogens have been used, synthesized either from 19-nortestosterone or from 17-α-hydroxyprogesterone. Derivatives of 19-nortestosterone are metabolised to a small extent to oestrogenic compounds, unlike the 17α-hydroxyprogesterone derivatives, and this may account for their powerful ovulation suppressant action. All of the marketed combination pills contain a 19-nortestosterone derivative plus an oestrogen. The 17α-hydroxyprogesterone derivative, medroxyprogesterone acetate, is used only in a progestogen-only contraceptive.

Table 15.1 Oestrogens and progestogens used in the contraceptive pill

Oestrogens	Progestogens
Ethinyloestradiol	**Derivatives of 19-nortestosterone**
	Norethynodrel
Mestranol (3-methyl	Norethisterone
ether of	Ethynodiol diacetate
ethinyloestradiol)	Lynoestrenol
	Norgestrel and levonorgestrel
	Derivatives of 17α-hydroxyprogesterone
	Medroxyprogesterone acetate

Mode of action

The oestrogenic compounds ethinyloestradiol and mestranol suppress ovulation by inhibiting the release of FSH from the anterior pituitary. In combination with a progestogen, particularly a 19-nortestosterone derivative, the antiovulatory effect largely accounts for the contraceptive action. Other changes take place, however, and contribute to this action. For instance, pseudo-decidual reactions occur in the endometrium and implantation of a fertilized ovum is impaired. The secretion of cervical mucus is reduced and it becomes thick and viscous so that spermatozoa are less able to penetrate into the uterine cavity. Furthermore, it is possible that the function of the corpus luteum might be disturbed by 17α-hydroxyprogesterone derivatives.

Progestogen-oestrogen combinations. These are usually taken for 21 or 22 days of the menstrual cycle, starting on the fifth day (counting from the onset of menstruation). A tablet-free interval of 6 or 7 days is then allowed, making a 28-day cycle. Withdrawal bleeding occurs during the tablet-free interval.

Sequential pills. These were developed in an attempt to achieve a more physiological control over ovulation. In the first part of the cycle, usually up to day 16 or 20, an oestrogen-only pill is taken, followed by a combined oestrogen-progestogen pill until day 25 or 26. A drug-free interval of 7 days is then allowed.

Low-dose progestogen-only pills. Concern over the adverse effects of oestrogen therapy has stimulated the development of pills containing only a progestogen in low dosage which is taken continuously. The contraceptive action of these pills is more limited, and ovulation can occur in up to 40% of cycles. Biochemical changes in cervical mucus probably account largely for the contraceptive action. This method cannot be recommended when a low failure rate is essential. Irregular menstrual bleeding is common. A depot preparation containing medroxyprogesterone acetate can be given intramuscularly and has a contraceptive action lasting for 3 months.

Minor adverse effects

The following occur commonly on starting the pill:

Nausea and occasional vomiting is common in the first cycle but usually settles in subsequent months. If it persists, a pregnancy test should be performed. Nausea is caused by the oestrogen component and a change to a less oestrogenic pill may help.

Breast tenderness and slight enlargement may occur during the first few cycles. It is an oestrogenic effect similar to that occurring in pregnancy.

Weight gain is common with some progestogenic preparations but is usually small and is lost after a few cycles.

Break-through bleeding, i.e. menstrual 'spotting' occurring in mid-cycle, is seen frequently at first especially with low-oestrogen pills and low-dose progestogen-only pills.

Post-pill amenorrhoea and hypofertility may occur, and can sometimes be prolonged.

Serious adverse effects

These, fortunately, occur rarely:

Thrombo-embolic disease. In the early 1960s, soon after the introduction of the contraceptive pill, reports began to appear of venous thrombo-embolism occurring in young women using the pill, and by 1966 a large number of case reports had appeared.

The results of formal epidemiological studies indicated that deep vein thrombosis and pulmonary embolism occurred more often than would be expected by chance alone in women taking the contraceptive pill. The relative risk was approximately 6–8 times greater in pill takers. The incidence correlates with both the dose of oestrogen and the dose of progestogen in the pill.

Ischaemic cerebrovascular disorders. The incidence of cerebral thrombosis is 5–6 times greater in women taking the pill. Cerebrovascular disease is normally rare in young women, which makes even more impressive the numbers of such cases reported in relationship to the contraceptive pill.

Assessment of the risk of thrombo-embolism associated with the use of the contraceptive pill requires consideration of a number of factors. The morbidity, and even the mortality, produced by other forms of contraception is not negligible and the risk of unwanted pregnancy may be higher than with the pill. Pregnancy itself causes an appreciable risk of complications, and legal abortion when unintended pregnancies occur is also not without hazard. It has been suggested that one oral contraceptive pill is as dangerous as smoking one-third of a cigarette once a day for 3 weeks out of 4.

In 1970, the Committee of Safety of Medicines considered that the evidence incriminating the oestrogen component of the contraceptive pill was strong enough to recommend that preparations containing no more than 50 μg of oestrogen should be used. Since this recommendation, the dose has been further reduced to 30 or 20 μg in some preparations, and there is evidence that this lessens the incidence of thrombo-embolic disease further. Low-dose progestogen-only pills seemed to be associated with a low risk, whereas sequential preparations produced a high risk.

Myocardial infarction. The incidence of pill taking in young women admitted to coronary care units is considerably higher than the expected incidence. In some women aged 40 or more on the combined pill, the risk of death from infarction approaches the incidence in males of a similar age.

Hypertension. Blood pressure is on average significantly increased by the contraceptive pill. Several high risk factors have been identified, such as obesity, a past history of toxaemia of pregnancy, and a family history of hypertension.

Jaundice. It is not surprising that oral contraceptives can cause jaundice, for many are 17α-alkyl-substituted steroids, and compounds of this type were known to be capable of causing cholestasis before the pill was introduced.

Haemangioma of liver. There is evidence of an increased incidence following long-term administration of the combined contraceptive pill.

Other adverse effects

The contraceptive pill has been held responsible for a number of other adverse effects, although in some cases the relationship has not been convincingly proven.

Depression, headaches and loss of libido occur frequently, but it must be remembered that these symptoms are common and should not always be put down to the pill.

Impairment of glucose tolerance can be caused by an effect on peripheral glucose metabolism, and occurs particularly in women with a family history of diabetes. Pre-existing diabetes may be worsened.

Fluid retention can occur, and care should be taken when prescribing for patients with renal or cardiac disease.

Intolerance to contact lenses has been reported.

Carcinogenic effects do not occur. In fact the incidence of some carcinomas, e.g. carcinoma of the cervix, may be reduced.

Interactions with the pill. These include interactions with liver enzyme inducers (see p. 18), and with broad-spectrum antibiotics such as amoxycillin which reduce their contraceptive effectiveness by interfering with enterohepatic cycling.

Conditions in which oestrogenic preparations should be avoided

A full medical examination is necessary before the pill is prescribed. Certain diseases are absolute contraindications to administration of oestrogenic preparations:

(i) Heart disease, and a previous history of thrombo-embolism. Caution may be necessary in a woman with hypertension.

(ii) Hepatic disease, including biliary cirrhosis, chronic active hepatitis, Dubin-Johnson and Rotor syndromes, and a history of idiopathic jaundice of pregnancy.

(iii) Cancers of the breast or genital tract.

(iv) Porphyria.

(v) Sickle cell anaemia.

16

Mild analgesics, anti-inflammatory drugs and corticosteroids

INFLAMMATION

The inflammatory reaction, both acute and chronic, is a basic defensive response to a variety of forms of injury. Some of the features of this reaction can be induced by a number of chemical mediators including kinins and histamine, but recent evidence suggests that prostaglandins may be of particular importance in many types of inflammation. They have been detected in exudates from experimentally induced inflammation, and abnormally high concentrations of prostaglandins E1, E2, F1α, and F2α were found when perfusion studies were carried out in the skin lesions of allergic volunteers with contact dermatitis.

Several different classes of drug possess anti-inflammatory properties and it has been difficult to define a mechanism of action common to them all. There is increasing evidence, however, that many of them interfere with prostaglandin activity. For example, aspirin, sodium salicylate, indomethacin and corticosteroids, in therapeutic concentrations, inhibit the synthesis of prostaglandins E2 and F2α from arachidonic acid by animal tissues. Fenamates (e.g. mefenamic acid) and aspirin block the bronchoconstrictor effects of prostaglandin F2α. It may be, therefore, that the anti-inflammatory drugs to the described possess in common the ability either to inhibit the synthesis or to block the activity of prostaglandins which mediate the inflammatory response.

Arachidonic acid may also be metabolized in the lung, platelets and white cells by lipid peroxidation catalyzed by the enzyme lipoxygenase. One product (HETE) is chemotactic for polymorphonuclear leucocytes and alveolar macrophages so these agents may be involved in the cellular invasion process of inflammation. A specific inhibitor of lipoxygenase is not available for human use so the therapeutic benefit of interruption of this pathway is still uncertain.

In diseases in which inflammation is the cause of pain, e.g. rheumatoid arthritis, it is logical to choose an analgesic drug with powerful anti-inflammatory activity, although drugs lacking this effect will nevertheless give satisfactory pain relief in mild disease. Many of the available analgesics have a central component to their therapeutic effect, although the relative contribution of such an action to the total drug effect may be difficult to determine.

MILD ANALGESICS AND ANTI-INFLAMMATORY DRUGS

The range of mild analgesics and anti-inflammatory drugs available is now wide. Aspirin is still the most widely used drug, however, and serves as a model non-steroidal anti-inflammatory (NSAID) drug with which to compare the newer preparations.

Salicylates

Although salicylates occur naturally, aspirin (acetylsalicylic acid) is a synthetic substance, and remains the most popular remedy for minor ailments, having displaced quinine from this position early in the present century. It is effective against headache, musculoskeletal pain and dysmenorrhea. It is readily absorbed after oral administration and 90% bound to plama proteins, particularly albumin, at therapeutic concentrations. Plasma protein binding is concentration-dependent, however, and falls to around 50% in overdose. Aspirin is rapidly converted during and after absorption to an active metabolite salicylic acid, so that its half-life is only 15 minutes. The half-life of salicylic acid is dose-dependent because of saturable metabolism and is around 2.5 hours after a 300 mg dose. As the dose is increased, clearance tends to fall and renal elimination of unchanged salicylic acid forms a larger proportion of the total body clearance of drug. Renal clearance of salicylic acid is pH dependent and increases with increasing alkalinity of the urine.

Aspirin is a powerful anti-inflammatory drug, having antihistamine, anti-5HT and anti-kinin properties, as well as inhibiting the synthesis of prostaglandins by inhibiting cyclo-oxygenase (page 158). It is anti-pyretic, probably acting directly on the hypothalamus, but despite this it increases the metabolic rate, and in overdosage can cause hyperpyrexia (see Ch. 21).

Gastrointestinal effects are the major adverse effects of aspirin.

Up to 70% of healthy subjects have occult blood in the faeces on taking therapeutic doses of aspirin. Dyspepsia occurs in a third of patients given aspirin in full doses for rheumatoid arthritis and it may also prolong the bleeding time. In larger doses it may reduce clotting factor synthesis and should not be prescribed for patients receiving anticoagulants. Because of these and other problems it should not be used for children under one year of age. Gastric complications are reduced by taking the dose after meals. Although the calcium salt ('soluble aspirin') is absorbed more quickly than the free acid, it causes a similar incidence of gastrointestinal effects. Enteric coated tablets may, however, reduce the gastrointestinal problems as will polymerised aluminium aspirin (aloxiprin) or micro-encapsulated preparations. Since these preparations are more slowly absorbed, they may be of less value in the treatment of short term pain, but are more suitable for chronic pain relief.

Diflunisal is a fluorinated salicylate with a longer half-life than aspirin, permitting twice daily administration. It appears to cause less gastrointestinal adverse effects than aspirin, but gastric haemorrhage has been described and, like salicylates, it can potentiate the action of warfarin and similar anticoagulants. Salicylate is hydrolysed after absorption to salicylic acid, and although producing fewer side effects, is otherwise similar to aspirin. Sodium salicylate is also similar to aspirin, although the latter is usually preferred. Each gram of sodium salicylate contains 6.25 m/moles of sodium, so it is contraindicated in the presence of severe renal disease or heart failure.

All salicylates can cause urticaria, vasomotor rhinitis and bronchospasm in susceptible individuals. These reactions are most common in females aged between 30 and 50, particularly in those with bronchial asthma who may also develop these effects after other non-steroidal anti-inflammatory agents. The effect may therefore be related to their cyclo-oxygenase inhibitory properties.

Paracetamol (Acetaminophen)

This is a widely used and effective analgesic for mild to moderate pain. It is the active metabolite of phenacetin which was withdrawn because of possible renal toxicity after long term administration. It is only a weak cyclo-oxygenase inhibitor, although it may be more effective against cyclo-oxygenase in the central nervous system than in the periphery. This may explain why although it is an effective analgesic and anti-pyretic, it has only weak anti-inflammatory activity at conventional doses. It is rapidly and completely absorbed from the gut, with peak levels 30 to 60 minutes after drug administration and a half-life in plasma of 1 to 4 hours at therapeutic doses. Virtually all of the drug is metabolized by conjugation in the liver. The incidence of adverse effects is low at normal doses, although it can cause hepatic and renal damage in overdose (see Ch. 20). Benorylate is a chemical combination of aspirin and paracetamol which is claimed to circumvent, at least in part, the gastric irritant properties of the salicylate moiety. Enzymatic cleavage in the liver breaks the chemical link. The adverse effects of benorylate resemble those of aspirin rather than those of paracetamol.

Fenamates

These include mefenamic acid and flufenamic acid. In addition to their anti-pyretic and anti-inflammatory effects they also seem to be effective in the treatment of primary spasmodic dysmenorrhoea. They can however cause severe diarrhoea in some individuals, as well as the other more common adverse effects of non-steroidal anti-inflammatory agents.

Propionic acid derivatives

Ibuprofen, ketoprofen, fenoprofen, naproxen and flurbiprofen are relatively weak antiflammatory agents but because of the relatively low incidence of adverse effects they are probably the drugs of first choice in musculo-skeletal and inflammatory joint disease. Ibuprofen seems to have the lowest incidence of adverse effects but it also a relatively weak agent. Fenbufen is a pro-drug, the active metabolites of which have long half-lives so it can be given on a once daily basis. Unlike the fenamates and pyrazolones, these agents do not inhibit the metabolism of warfarin.

Phenylacetic acid derivatives

These have potencies similar to the propionic acid derivatives. Fenclofenac can cause skin rashes in 25% of patients given the drug and although rashes are not so frequent with diclofenac, gastrointestinal intolerance is a greater problem.

Indole derivatives

Indomethacin has been used for many years and is very effective. It can be used in high doses for short periods of time, e.g. in the treatment of acute exacerbations of gout: in a single large dose last thing at night to prevent early morning stiffness in rheumatoid arthritis; or daily in divided doses for relief of chronic inflammatory joint disease. Large doses appear to reasonably well tolerated for short periods of time, but chronic use is associated with a high incidence of CNS complications, particularly headache and dizziness, and more rarely drowsiness, confusion and depression. Gastrointestinal upset and bleeding are also more frequent than with some other agents. Sulindac is better tolerated and can be given on a twice daily basis, but is less effective than indomethacin. Tolmetin is probably as potent as indomethacin but is better tolerated.

Pyrazolone derivates

Although phenylbutazone and its derivative oxyphenbutazone are potent anti-inflammatory drugs with urocosuric activity, their use is limited by the high incidence of adverse effects which they produce, particularly on the gastrointestinal and central nervous systems and the skin. The more serious adverse effects are on the bone marrow with thrombocytopaenia, agranulocytosis and aplastic anaemia, (occasionally fatal) which occurs in about 1 in 8000 administrations. Phenylbutazone appears to cause fluid retention more commonly than other non-steroidal anti-inflammatory drugs and may precipitate cardiac failure. They also inhibit the metabolism of warfarin and tolbutamide. Oxyphenbutazone has now been withdrawn and phenylbutazone is only used for the treatment of severe ankylosing spondylitis and then only in the hospital situation where regular haematological monitoring is possible. Azapropazone, although less effective, is better tolerated and has no tendency to cause blood dyscrasias, although rashes may occur. Like the other pyrazolones, azapropazone inhibits warfarin metabolism and can potentiate its anticoagulant action markedly.

Piroxicam

Piroxicam is a relatively new agent with a long elimination half-life so it can be given as a single daily dose. It may produce gastrointestinal problems and may cause more fluid retention than some other agents so it should be used with caution in the elderly.

RENAL EFFECTS OF NON-STEROIDAL ANTI-INFLAMATORY AGENTS AND OTHER WEAK ANALGESICS

Prostaglandins produced in the kidney regulate renal blood flow and glomerular filtration rate, particularly when renal perfusion pressure is already low. It is therefore not surprising that NSAIDs may produce deleterious effects on the kidney. They may promote renal sodium, water and potassium retention, particularly in patients with borderline cardiac and renal failure.

Acute renal failure caused by NSAIDs has also been described in patients in whom renal perfusion pressure has been reduced by other factors such as depletion of the extracellular fluid volume by shock, surgical stress, haemorrhage or concurrent diuretic therapy. It can occur in otherwise healthy subjects after overdose of NSAIDs however and is associated with acute tubular necrosis which normally responds to drug withdrawal.

Acute interstitial nephritis leading to proteinuria and the nephrotic syndrome has also been reported, particularly with the propionic acid derivatives (especially fenoprofen). It is a dose-independent phenomenon and the mechanism is unknown, although it normally resolves gradually after drug withdrawal. NSAIDs can occasionally cause a glomerulonephritis associated with a systemic vasculitis, but this is also normally reversed by drug discontinuation. Finally, renal papillary necrosis has been associated with NSAID use. This may be the mechanism of the nephropathy seen in patients who have consumed analgesics (often in mixtures containing several different agents) for long periods. There are striking geographical differences in the incidence of the nephropathy which are related relatively closely to differences in consumption of analgesic mixtures. Although no single agent has been incriminated, patients should be discouraged from unnecessary chronic ingestion of any mild analgesic, whether alone or contained in a mixture.

GOUT

Gout is a metabolic disorder caused by an inborn error of uric acid metabolism, which produces attacks of painful arthritis and, in advanced stages, deposition of urate crystals in joints, subcutaneous tissues, kidneys and heart.

Treatment of the acute attack

Indomethacin in relatively high dose, or one of the other non-steroidal anti-inflammatory agents (e.g. azapropazone) is normally given for immediate pain relief. Colchicine is effective, but has a high incidence of nausea, vomiting and diarrhoea associated with its use. It is now generally only used in those who are unable to tolerate non-steroidal anti-inflammatory drugs.

Prophylatic treatment

(a) *Allopurinol.* The formation of uric acid from xanthine and hypoxanthine is catalyzed by the enzyme xanthine oxidase. Allopurinol, which resembles hypoxanthine structurally, inhibits this enzyme and so reduces uric acid formation so that serum uric acid falls. Urate deposits may also be reduced. Allopurinol is effective not only in primary gout but also in other conditions in which there is excessive production of uric acid, such as polycythaemia and the leukaemias. Since its activity lies in the metabolite, oxypurinol, which has a long half-life, it can usually be given in single daily doses unless the total daily amount exceeds 300 mg per day. It should only be given once the acute episode has subsided and a non-steroidal anti-inflammatory agent should be continued for around 2 months in low dose as prophylaxis against acute attacks. The most common adverse effect is skin rash, particularly in patients with chronic renal failure and the dose should be reduced in this condition. Allopurinol inhibits the metabolism of azathiaprine and 6-mercaptopurine and the dose of these two drugs should be reduced in patients receiving allopurinol.

(b) *Uricosuric drugs* such as probenecid, sulphinpyrazone and azapropazone inhibit the active reabsorption of uric acid by the proximal renal tubule. The uricosuric effects are greatly reduced when the creatinine clearance drops below 50 ml per minute so they are less useful in patients with renal failure. Patients should maintain a high fluid intake, especially in the first few weeks of treatment to ensure that an adequate urine output protects against crystallization of uric acid in the kidney. Alkalinization of the urine may also protect against this problem. Sulphinpyrazone and probenecid are the most widely used uricosuric agents. Both drugs cause occasional nausea and vomiting and hypersensitivity reactions and blood dyscrasias have been rarely described. Allopurinol has largely replaced uricosuric agents for prophylactic treatment of gout.

OTHER DRUGS USED IN RHEUMATOID ARTHRITIS

Although non-steroidal anti-inflammatory agents provide symptomatic relief in rheumatic diseases, they appear not to modify the course of the disease. If this appears to be progressive, particularly in the presence of erosive arthritis, second-line drugs are necessary, such as gold, penicillamine, hydroxychloroquine and sulphasalazine. None of these drugs produce an immediate effect and it may take up to 6 months to achieve the full benefits of therapy. They may also improve the extra-articular manifestations of the disease.

Gold salts

Gold salts appear to be of value in the treatment of some patients with active rheumatoid arthritis and juvenile chronic arthritis (Still's disease). The agent is given as a weekly intramuscular dose of sodium aurothiomalate. This is gradually increased in dose over the first 4 weeks and the patient is carefully observed for adverse effects including blood dyscrasias, proteinuria, stomatitis, hepatitis and pulmonary fibrosis. If no response has been seen when 1 g of gold has been given, another agent should be tried. If response does occur, a small maintenance dose at less frequent intervals may prevent relapse. If relapse occurs, it should be treated immediately by increasing the dose of gold.

Penicillamine

Penicillamine is a powerful metal chelator, although its mode of action in rheumatoid arthritis is unknown. It may be an even more effective disease modifying agent than gold, particularly on the extra articular manifestations of the disease. The dose of the drug is increased gradually but if no response has occurred after a year it is discontinued. The adverse effects appear to be related to the dose and include blood dyscrasias, particularly thrombocytopaenia, and a myasthenic syndrome, proteinurea, skin rashes and systemic lupus erythematosus-like syndrome. The drug has also been used to increase copper elimination in Wilson's disease (hepatolenticular degeneration) and in chronic active hepatitis, primary biliary cirrhosis and cystinuria.

Antimalarial drugs

Chloroquine and its close relative hydroxychloroquine appear to possess anti-inflammatory properties, although the mechanism is unknown. They have been used in the treatment of rheumatoid arthritis, discoid lupus erythematosus and systemic lupus erythematosus. 70% of the drug is excreted unchanged in the urine and the half-life of the parent compound in plasma is around one week. Both agents are approximately as effective as gold but have fewer adverse effects. Toxicity involving the cornea and retina is a major problem which may be irreversible. Retinopathy is more common in the elderly and the drug is best avoided by patients over 55 years of age, but is also related to the dose and duration of treatment which should be kept to a minimum.

Immunosuppressive agents

Azathioprine and chlorambucil have both been used in patients with rheumatoid arthritis who have failed to respond to other second-line disease modifying agents. They are also used in other progressive and potentially fatal inflammatory conditions in which it is believed that an autoimmune mechanism is at work, such as systemic lupus-erythematosus, particularly in the presence of severe renal disease. It is not certain, however, whether the therapeutic benefit sometimes achieved is due to suppression of specific immune mechanisms or to non-specific anti-inflammatory effects. Immunosuppressants have also been used in polymyositis which has not responded adequately to steroids alone and in this, and other chronic inflammatory conditions, they may exert a steroid-sparing effect, thus reducing the incidence of long term toxicity of corticosteroids.

Cyclosporin, a polypeptide obtained from soil fungi, inhibits T lymphocyte proliferation and cell mediated immunity. Although not used in rheumatoid arthritis it appears to be effective in preventing organ rejection after transplantation and may also have effects in autoimmune disease. Although it is not myelotoxic, it is nephrotoxic and hepatotoxic and may cause hirsutism and gastrointestinal disturbances.

Corticosteroids

Steroid hormones secreted by the adrenal cortex may be subdivided into: (a) glucocorticoids, such as hydrocortisone and cortisone which exert their chief effect on fat, protein and carbohydrate metabolism and possess marked anti-inflammatory activity; and (b) mineralocorticoids, such desoxycorticosterone and aldosterone, which are concerned primarily with electrolyte and water balance. In addition to their glucocorticoid effects, hydrocortisone and cortisone both have marked mineralocorticoid actions, which are a disadvantage when they are being used as anti-inflammatory agents. Newer synthetic steroids have fewer such actions.

Cortisone was originally isolated from adrenal extracts but is now synthesized for therapeutic use. It is rapidly hydroxylated to hydro-cortisone (cortisol) by the liver, and is used only for replacement therapy in Addison's disease. Hydrocortisone is believed to be the most important naturally secreted glucocorticoid hormone of the adrenal cortex. Prednisolone, prednisone (which is hydroxylated to prednisolone after absorption), triamcinolone, dexamethasone and betamethasone possess greater anti-inflammatory properties without an increase in salt retaining activity (see Table 16.1).

Table 16.1   Relative glucocorticoid and mineralocorticoid activity of some corticosteroid drugs

	Relative anti-inflammatory activity (glucocorticoid)	Relative salt-retaining potency (mineralocorticoid)
Cortisone	1	1
Hydrocortisone	1	1
Prednisone	5	1
Prednisolone	5	1
Triamcinolone	5	< 1
Dexamethasone	35	< 1
Betamethasone	35	< 1

Corticosteroids demonstrate the following actions:

(a) Atrophy of the adrenal cortex, with the exception of the zona glomerulosa, and depression of normal adrenal cortical function. This is due to suppression of release of adrenocorticotrophic hormone from the pituitary gland, due in turn to suppression of corticotrophin-releasing factor from the hypothalamus.

(b) Retention of sodium and increased loss of potassium from the body. Adrenal cortical insufficiency is associated with sodium loss, hyponatraemia, hyperkalaemia, and a reduction in the extracellular fluid volume. These changes are reversed by adrenal steroid hormones, particularly the mineralocorticoids such as aldosterone. In the normal subject sodium retention leads to increased body weight, hypertension and oedema.

(c) Increased gluconeogenesis through mobilization of protein and amino acids from skeletal muscle.

(d) Shrinkage of lymphoid tissue and reduction in lymphocyte production leading to a lymphocytopenia in the blood.

(e) Reduction in the blood eosinophil count and rise in the neutrophil granulocyte count.

(f) Suppression of the inflammatory response.

The clinical indications for systemic treatment with corticosteroids are:

1. Replacement therapy in patients with adrenal cortical insufficiency due to Addison's disease, the Waterhouse-Friderichsen syndrome or post-adrenalectomy. It is usual to combine treatment with a synthetic mineralocorticoid compound such as fludrocortisone with cortisone. The salt retaining activity of prednisolone or one of the other synthetic glucocorticoids is not sufficient for satisfactory replacement therapy.

2. Treatment with pharmacological doses of steroids.

(a) Shrinkage of lymphatic tissue and suppression of lymphopoiesis in patients with leukaemias and lymphomas.

(b) Suppression of the rejection phenomenon in tissue transplantation.

(c) Anti-inflammatory therapy in a variety of conditions including rheumatoid arthritis, systemic lupus erythematosus, polyarteritis, dermatomyositis, ulcerative colitis, sarcoidosis, the nephrotic syndrome, bronchial asthma, severe inflammatory conditions of the eye and skin, cerebral oedema and raised intracranial pressure. Corticosteroids are also used in the treatment of autoimmune haemolytic anaemia and thrombocytopenic purpura.

For replacement therapy cortisone, hydrocortisone and fludrocortisone are the preparations of choice. For the treatment of leukaemia, lymphoma and inflammatory conditions steroids with more potent effects but with relatively less salt-retaining properties are used, particularly prednisolone or prednisone. As prednisone is converted to prednisolone after absorption, it is rational to regard prednisolone as the standard drug of choice for these indications. It may be administered orally, intravenously, by enema, intra-articularly, or locally to the eye and skin. The more potent steroids dexamethasone and betamethasone are used where very high doses are required to suppress the inflammatory reaction or other disease process, and in local conditions of the eye and skin. Dexamethasone is used to suppress the adrenal cortex in tests of pituitary-adrenal function and to reduce raised intracranial pressure caused by brain oedema associated with, for example, brain tumour or status epilepticus. Beclamethasone and budesonide are used by inhalation or nebulization for the treatment of asthma in order to reduce the risk of adverse effects.

Adverse effects of corticosteroid therapy

The following complications of corticosteroid therapy may be seen, particularly in the high doses required for anti-inflammatory activity. They are not seen in replacement doses for adrenocortical insufficienty.

1. Fulminating infections. The normal inflammatory responses to bacterial and viral infection are reduced or masked. Latent tuberculous foci may be reactivated.

2. Osteoporosis and collapse of vertebrae due to mobilization of tissue proteins in gluconeogenesis.

3. Myopathy with muscle weakness and wasting, especially involving the proximal girdle muscles. This is especially prominent with triamcinolone.

4. Diabetes mellitus due to gluconeogenesis and increased insulin resistance.

5. Hypertension, due to sodium and water retention. This may proceed to cardiac failure.

6. Weight gain, oedema, bruising, purple striae in the skin particularly of the abdomen, moon face.

7. Psychotic reactions of all types may occur.

8. Hirsutism and menstrual disturbances.

9. Pancreatitis.

10. Cataracts may be seen after long-term treatment.

11. Retardation of growth may be seen after long term use in children.

12. Withdrawal phenomena. The adrenal suppression accompanying steroid therapy leads to symptoms and signs of adrenal insufficiency if the steroid is abruptly withdrawn. These are anorexia, nausea, vomiting, diarrhoea, abdominal pain, headache, arthralgia, restlessness, lethargy, muscle weakness, temperature disturbances, dehydration, hypotension and vascular collapse. The

condition is treated with saline infusion and administration or fludrocortisone and hydrocortisone. Doses should always be gradually reduced to avoid acute adrenal insufficiency.

Therapeutic use of corticosteroids has been thought either to cause peptic ulceration, or to prevent established ulcers from healing. Adverse effects can be reduced by using intermittent therapy, (e.g. in exacerbations of asthma), or by keeping chronic doses as low as possible, and on occasion by using them in a single higher dose on alternate days (in the evening) rather than daily.

Interactions involving corticosteroids (see p. 37)

Corticotrophins

Corticotrophin (adrenocorticotrophic hormone) is a polypeptide secreted by the anterior pituitary gland under the influence of corticotrophin-releasing factor from the hypothalamus. It stimulates the adrenal cortex to secrete hydrocortisone and other hormones, and is administered parenterally by intramuscular or intravenous injection as its activity is rapidly destroyed by proteolytic enzymes in the gastrointestinal tract. Long-acting preparations of corticotrophin in gelatin solution or adsorbed on to zinc hydroxide are available for daily intramuscular injection.

Synthetic corticotrophic hormones which consist of part of the peptide chain of natural corticotrophin have been prepared, for example, tetracosactrin. They are preferable for use in patients who show hypersensitivity to natural corticotrophin, although hypersensitivity reactions to the synthetic agent have been described, albeit rarely. There is evidence that it may be absorbed through the nasal mucosa when administered as snuff.

Corticotrophins may be used in those conditions for which corticosteroids are given, apart from adrenal cortical replacement therapy. Such treatment involves regular injections, however, which is less convenient particularly in long-term therapy, and most physicians prefer to use oral corticosteroids. In children corticotrophin may be preferable because there is evidence that it retards growth less than corticosteroids. Adrenal suppression does not follow the use of corticotrophin as it does with corticosteroids, and patients treated with it tend to retain a normal adrenal response to stress. Hypertension, pigmentation, hirsutism and acne occur more frequently as complications of corticotrophin therapy because it stimulates the production of androgenic steroids as well as cortisol.

Dyspepsia, bruising, striae formation, osteoporosis and myopathy are less frequent with corticotrophin.

ANTIHISTAMINES

Histamine receptors can be subdivided into H1- and H2-receptors. The latter are found in the stomach and atria, and are not blocked by the traditional antihistamine drugs. The account which follows is confined to the traditional H1 antihistamines. H2-receptor antagonists are discussed in Ch. 12.

The number of proprietary antihistamine preparations is enormous, but, as is usual in these circumstances, there are only minor differences between them. It is an easy matter to produce a useful antihistamine, which is the reason why most drug companies market at least one. Antihistamine properties are ubiquitous among compounds belonging to other pharmacological groups, including phenothiazine tranquillisers, antidepressants and α-adrenergic blocking drugs. Likewise, antihistamines have many other pharmacological actions (Table 16.2). Briefly their pharmacology can be summarized as follows:

Table 16.2   Relative sedative, anticholinergic and anti-emetic properties of some antihistamines.

	Sedative effect	Anticholinergic effect	Anti-emetic effect	Other uses
Promethazine	+++	+++	++	Sedative, hypnotic, anti-emetic
Diphenhydramine	+++	+++	++	
Cyproheptadine	++	++	Minimal	Appetite stimulant 5HT antagonist
Cyclizine	+	+	+++	Anti-emetic
Astemizole	Minimal	Minimal	Minimal	
Terfenadine	Minimal	Minimal	Minimal	
Ketotifen	+	+	Not evaluated	Prophylaxis of asthma

(a) Antihistamine effect. This is a competitive antagonism, and must be contrasted with the physiological reversal of histamine actions by adrenaline. Although the bronchoconstrictor and vasodilator effects of histamine are antagonized, the histamine-induced gastric acid production, mediated through H2 receptors, is not inhibited.

(b) Anticholinergic properties. These produce peripheral atrophine-like adverse effects, such as dryness of the mouth, blurred vision and tachycardia. They may account also for the value of some antihistamines as anti-emetic and anti-Parkinsonian drugs, although one of the most powerful anti-emetics, cyclizine, has weak peripheral atropine-like effects. Diphenhydramine has been used in Parkinsonism, but its effects are mild compared with those of other anticholinergics. Antihistamines with marked anticholinergic actions, such as diphenhydramine and promethazine, should not be given to patients with glaucoma or prostatic hypertrophy.

(c) α-adrenergic and 5HT blocking actions are possessed particularly by the phenothiazine derivative promethazine. Cyproheptadine, related structurally to imipramine, has potent anti-5HT effects, and has been used to antagonize the peripheral effects of 5HT secreted by carcinoid tumours. It stimulates appetite.

(d) Local anaesthetic actions. This is most marked with antazoline, which has been used as an antiarrhythmic.

(e) Central effects. Sedation is one of the main drawbacks of most antihistamines, and the major effort in the development of these compounds has been concentrated on producing a non-sedative drug. Promethazine and diphenhydramine are the worst from this point of view, although this is of value when the former drug is used as a long acting hypnotic. Astemizole and terfenadine are generally considered to be better in this respect than most antihistamines. Patients should be advised to avoid alcohol and other central depressant drugs, whose actions are increased by antihistamines, and drivers should be warned of these effects. Despite their sedative properties some antihistamines have convulsant properties and should not, if possible, be used by epileptics.

(f) Other actions. Topical use of these drugs can cause photosensitivity and other skin eruptions, and should be avoided. Gastrointestinal disturbances occur occasionally, including epigastric distress, anorexia, nausea and constipation or diarrhoea. Agranulocytosis, haemolytic anaemia and thrombocytopenia occur rarely. Cyclizine is possibly teratogenic, and should therefore be avoided by women of child-bearing age.

Indications for use

Antihistamines are of most value when histamine plays a major role in the clinical syndrome produced by an immune reaction. This is the case in acute allergic responses to drugs, chemicals, certain foodstuffs and pollen, producing acute urticarial reactions and seasonal hay-fever. These conditions are considerably relieved by oral administration of an antihistamine and withdrawal, if possible, of the allergen. A generalized anaphylactic reaction requires more urgent action, and here administration of subcutaneous adrenaline is essential. Antihistamines are only of supplementary benefit, partly because other substances, e.g. various kinins, may be involved in this reaction. Similarly, angioneurotic oedema is better treated with adrenaline, for although it is improved by antihistamines they do not act quickly enough in a life-threatening situation.

Pruritus is relieved only when it is caused by histamine release, as in the itching accompanying acute urticaria, and following insect bites. If the lesions are localized, application of antihistamine ointment are of some value, but repeated and extensive use should be discouraged because of the risk of photosensitivity. Pruritus not caused by histamine release is better treated by a phenothiazine. Chronic urticaria and chronic allergies, (e.g. contact dermatitis), are less often helped. Similarly, antihistamines are of little value in serum sickness, although accompanying urticarial skin lesions may be improved.

Bronchial asthma does not respond to oral or intravenous antihistamines, even when there is an obvious allergic cause such as pollen sensitivity. The only exception to this is bronchospasm from the release of histamine by drugs, such as dextran and tubocurarine, although even in this case adrenaline is more effective. The course of a common cold is not influenced by antihistamine, although their atropine-like effects may reduce nasal secretions to some extent. The use of antihistamines as anti-emetics is discussed on page 107.

Choice of drug

The main consideration in choosing an antihistamine is whether or not sedation is desirable. Occasionally it is, as for instance in an acute-urticarial reaction or for a patient who is being kept awake by itching. But in most cases it is undesirable, e.g. for a patient who continues to work or drive while receiving an antihistamine for hayfever. There is considerable variation in response to the various antihistamines. One patient may be sedated by one drug, whereas another patient is not. It is therefore worthwhile trying several drugs for patients who will need prolonged administration.

17

Vitamins and iron

Vitamins are essential constituents of the diet because, excepting vitamin D and nicotinic acid, they cannot be synthesized in the body. Vitamins B and C are water soluble, whereas vitamins A, D and K are fat soluble and likely to be malabsorbed in steatorrhoea. Although the consumption of vitamin preparations is enormous, the clinical indications for their administration are few.

Vitamin A

Dietary vitamin A comes from animal sources, particularly liver and dairy produce, and from certain vegetables such as carrots and tomatoes. Margarine is reinforced with vitamins A and D. The daily requirement is about 2500 iu, with a higher intake during pregnancy and lactation. In Britain deficiency of this vitamin is rare, and is almost always associated with malabsorption and steatorrhea, but in some underdeveloped countries it is common.

Vitamin A has two essential functions, (a) it is a constituent part of visual purple (rhodopsin); and (b) it plays an important part in the maintenance of epithelial surfaces. Severe deficiency of the vitamin can cause a defect in dark adaptation, leading to night blindness, and conversion of mucous surfaces into stratified squamous epithelium. When the cornea and conjunctiva are involved xerophthalmia and keratomalacia can occur if the condition remains untreated.

For treatment of deficiency disease 50 000 iu should be administered daily until the symptoms have resolved. Prophylactic vitamin A, usually in conjunction with vitamin D, is often given to pregnant and lactating women, and to infants. Chronic ingestion of large quantities of the vitamin can produce toxicity, manifested by irritability, loss of appetite, itching and hypoprothrombinaemia. Peeling of the skin can occur in acute intoxication, as occurred in Arctic explorers who ate polar bear liver.

Vitamin B group

Four vitamins of this group will be dealt with together because a deficiency of one is usually accompanied by a deficiency of the others, and clinical syndromes are often mixed. These include thiamine hydrochloride (aneurine, B_1), riboflavine (B_2), pyridoxine (B_6) and nicotinic acid (B_7). Folic acid and cyanocobalamin (B_{12}) are dealt with separately below.

Thiamine is of importance as a coenzyme in the decarboxylation of pyruvic acid. The clinical deficiency syndrome includes cardiac failure (wet beri-beri), peripheral neuritis (dry beri-beri) and Wernicke's encephalopathy (cerebral beri-beri). It is a disease of under-developed countries, but is occassionally seen in Britain, particularly in alcoholics. Cardiac beri-beri usually responds dramatically to administration of physiological amounts of thiamine, and the the diagnosis is probably often overlooked, for a normal ward diet contains sufficient of the B vitamins to overcome the deficiency in a few days. Neurological forms of the disease respond more slowly, especially the peripheral neuritis, probably because factors other than thiamine deficiency are involved.

Riboflavine acts as a coenzyme for a variety of respiratory enzymes. Its deficiency leads to angular stomatitis and ulceration of mucous membranes, but is usually accompanied by other B vitamin deficiency diseases. In Britain angular stomatitis is usually caused by factors other than riboflavine deficiency.

Pyridoxine is converted to pyridoxal phosphate in the body and acts as a coenzyme to transaminases. Pyridoxine deficiency can cause fits in infancy. Rarely, familial pyridoxine resistance occurs. Large doses of pyridoxine are sometimes of value in sideroblastic anaemia, which is a type of hypochromic anaemia in which the adequate stores of iron in the bone marrow cannot be incorporated into red cells.

Nicotinic acid is an essential component of co-dehydrogenases I and II. Deficiency of this vitamin causes pellagra, with its classical trio of symptoms, dermatitis, dementia and diarrhoea. It is extremely rare in Britain, although it is occasionally seen in patients with disturbed tryptophan metabolism (e.g. during isoniazid therapy) for nicotinic acid is normally synthesized endogenously from tryptophan as well as being absorbed from the diet. Nicotinic acid can cause flushing of the blush areas when used in large doses to treat hypercholesterolaemia.

Indications for use

The use of these four vitamins, either alone, or in a multi-vitamin preparation is indicated only in a few well defined circumstances.

(*a*) *Dietary deficiency.* The average diet of the British population contains generous amounts of these vitamins and therefore the use of tonics and other preparations containing them is entirely unnecessary in a healthy person receiving a normal diet. Intake can become critical or frankly inadequate in two types of person, the alcoholic and the elderly person living alone. Obviously the best treatment is to ensure an adequate diet, but the use of vitamin supplements has a place, particularly in the immediate treatment of a clinical deficiency. For this purpose a parenteral multivitamin preparation (Parenterovite) is generally used.

(*b*) *Malabsorption.* Deficiency of the B vitamins is unusual in malabsorption, but supplements are occasionally necessary when treatment fails to control the malabsorptive state.

(*c*) *Prolonged vomiting and intravenous feeding.* Parenteral treatment with B vitamins may be necessary in hyperemesis gravidarum, gastrointestinal disease or following major surgery.

(*d*) *Antibiotic treatment.* Isoniazid can interfere with the metabolism of pyridoxine and can cause peripheral neuritis when prolonged courses are given, as is usual when the drug is used for treating tuberculosis. It occurs only when the serum level of the drug is excessive, as in slow acetylators. Prophylactic pyridoxine may be necessary when higher doses of isoniazid are given. The adverse effects of tetracline administration, such as sore mouth and diarrhoea, are not the result of vitamin deficiency.

Folic acid

In contrast to the other vitamins of the B group, deficiency of folic acid is relatively common. Although severe deficiency can cause megaloblastic anaemia, there is some evidence that a milder deficiency can produce more general symptoms such as malaise and anorexia, but no adequately controlled studies have been performed. There may also be a connection between folate deficiency and certain obstetric complications and fetal abnormalities.

Serum and red cell levels of folate can be readily measured with microbiological assays. The red cell level is more representative of the tissue stores of folate than the serum level, which fluctuates with dietary intake. The daily requirement of an adult is about 50–75 μg, and the average diet contains two or three times this amount. In the last trimester of pregnancy, however, the physiological requirement is increased to 150–200 μg/day and therefore a deficiency can easily occur when the diet is below standard. Mild folate deficiency is so common in pregnancy that it is standard practice in most obstetric units to prescribe a folic acid supplement. Other causes of folate deficiency are malabsorption, certain diseases in which folate requirements are increased, such as malignancy, leukaemias, chronic inflammatory conditions and psoriasis, and certain substances which interfere with folate metabolism, such as anticonvulsant drugs, nitrofurantoin and folic acid antagonists.

Indications for use

There are two indications for administration of folic acid, (a) to treat established deficiency and (b) as prophylaxis in conditions known to be associated with an increased requirement for the vitamin.

(a) Established deficiency is treated with 5–15 mg of folic acid (pteroylmonoglutamic acid) daily to replete body stores. The subsequent maintenance dose depends upon the body requirement. This seldom exceeds 300 μg/day, but in practice much larger doses are given. Up to 50% of patients on anticonvulsant drugs have low folate levels, but megaloblastic anaemia is rare. There is little evidence that replacement therapy helps in any way in the absence of megaloblastic anaemia.

Folic acid should never be given alone when the serum level of vitamin B_{12} is low, as in Addisonian pernicious anaemia, because neurological complications can be precipitated despite haematological improvement. Physiological doses (100 μg) of folic acid are often used as a therapeutic trial to confirm the cause of a patient's megaloblastic anaemia.

(b) Prophylaxis in pregnancy is justified by the frequency with which haematological evidence of anaemia occurs, and by the possible role of folate deficiency in causing obstetric complications. It is usual to give a combined iron and folic acid preparation, although the optimum dose of each is a matter of dispute. Proprietary preparations contain from 100 μg to 5 mg of folic acid and 30 to 150 mg of iron.

Treatment with cytostatic folic acid antagonists may produce signs of folate deficiency for which folinic acid may be required.

Vitamin B$_{12}$

The average daily intake of vitamin B$_{12}$ is 5–10 μg and this is greatly in excess of the body requirement. Dietary deficiency is therefore rare. Clinical deficiency disease is seen when there is malabsorption due to lack of intrinsic factor (pernicious anaemia), following total or partial gastrectomy, or in various small bowel diseases. The effects of vitamin B$_{12}$ deficiency are megaloblastic anaemia, peripheral neuropathy and subacute combined degeneration of the spinal cord, and dementia. Administration of the vitamin is indicated in several circumstances.

(a) Established deficiency, of whatever cause, should be treated with several injections of 1000 μg at intervals of a few days between each injection in order to replete the liver stores of the vitamin. Maintenance doses of 250 μg/month are more than adequate to meet the daily requirement. In megaloblastic anaemia caused by vitamin B$_{12}$ deficiency a brisk reticulocyte response is seen, reaching a peak at about 7 days after the start of treatment. A single dose as small as 100 ng is enough to produce a reticulocyte response, and this can be a useful diagnostic test. Improvement of neurological lesions is slow and often incomplete.

(b) Prophylaxis is given in patients who will, or might, become deficient as a result of gastric surgery. This is an inevitable result of total gastrectomy.

(c) Leber's optic atrophy and tobacco amblyopia respond to large doses of vitamin B$_{12}$.

Vitamin B$_{12}$ is available as cyanocobalamin or hydroxocobalamin. The latter is the more satisfactory preparation as it is retained in the body more readily.

Vitamin C (ascorbic acid)

The main function of this vitamin is the conversion of proline to hydroxyproline, which is an important constituent of collagen and intercellular substance. When it is lacking intercellular substance becomes thin and watery, giving little support to blood vessels in tissues, and as a result petichial haemorrhages and ecchymoses occur. The gums become inflamed and swollen. Lack of collagen in bone causes easy fracturing and poor healing. Anaemia, of either a macrocytic or normocytic type, can occur. This clinical syndrome is called scurvy.

The daily requirement is 20–30 mg/day, but scurvy does not

occur unless the daily intake is below 10 mg for many months. Deficiency is rare, and is confined to the elderly and the very young. The vitamin is found exclusively in fruit and vegetables, the potato being the main dietary source. Many fruit drinks are supplemented with vitamin C. A high intake results in a high urinary excretion.

Indication for use

Administration of vitamin C is necessary only when deficiency has been diagnosed or, prophylactically, when the diet is deficient in the vitamin, e.g. in infants and the elderly. Patients with a subclinical deficiency show delayed healing of wounds after surgery, and for this reason some surgeons prescribe the vitamin routinely. It is often used in the common cold and other infections, although the evidence that it promotes recovery is equivocal.

Vitamin D

Included under this name are several steroid compounds which have antirachitic properties. Vitamin D_2 (ergocalciferol) is derived by ultraviolet irradiation of a provitamin (ergosterol) of vegetable origin and is the most widely used clinically. Dihydrotachysterol is derived from the same provitamin. Vitamin D_3 (cholecalciferol) is produced by irradiation of 7-dehydrocholesterol, a provitamin of animal origin which is found in the Malpighian layer of the human skin, and which is converted to cholecalciferol by sunlight. This vitamin is found also in milk and fish liver oils, and is added to margarine.

The antirachitic activity of these vitamins is dependent upon their conversion into active metabolites by hydroxylation in the liver and kidneys (Fig. 17.1). 25-Hydroxycholecalciferol is produced in the liver, and this is further hydroxylated to 1,25-dihydroxycholecalciferol by the kidneys. These are the chief active metabolites. Other more polar metabolites are produced, but are biologically inactive. Anticonvulsant drugs interfere with hepatic hydroxylation, leading to accelerated production of inactive metabolites. Renal disease can impair the production of the dihydroxy derivative. In both these situations osteomalacia can occur.

Rickets in childhood results from an inadequate dietary intake and lack of exposure to sunlight, and was common in the industrial cities of Victorian England. Familial vitamin D resistance is

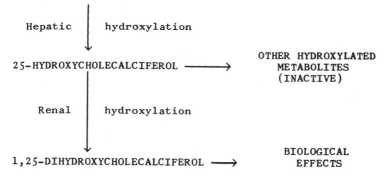

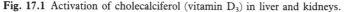

Fig. 17.1 Activation of cholecalciferol (vitamin D₃) in liver and kidneys.

occasionally seen. In adults, deficiency can result from disease of the biliary tract or intestine, for vitamin D is fat soluble and will be lost when steatorrhoea exists.

Vitamin D promotes the intestinal absorption of calcium and phosphorous, their mobilization from bone and possibly their renal excretion. Serum calcium levels are increased, and hypercalcaemia can occur with overdosage, producing renal calcinosis and renal failure. The metabolic effects of vitamin D and parathormone are closely interrelated.

A daily intake of 10 μg (400 iu) is adequate during childhood, pregnancy and lactation. In adults 5 μg is probably adequate, but the average diet contains considerably greater amounts than this. Exposure to sunlight has a potent antirachitic effect.

Indications for use

(a) Treatment of rickets and osteomalacia. Physiological doses will promote rapid healing when the diet has been deficient. In practice up to 250 μg daily are given, but it is important to avoid too high a dose. Renal calcinosis can occur with chronic intake of 1 mg daily. When bone disease has been caused by bowel disease, renal disease or familial vitamin D resistance much larger doses may be required, up to 10 mg daily. Frequent estimation of the serum calcium level is necessary. 1α-Hydroxycholecalciferol (alfacalcidol) has been synthesized and appears to be particularly useful in osteomalacia due to renal disease, in which the 1-hydroxylase mechanism is impaired. It has a rapid onset of effect and is useful in the early management of patients with symptoms of hypocalcaemia. Overdosage can occur with prolonged use, but stopping treatment soon reverses the metabolic changes.

(b) Treatment of hypoparathyroidism. Parathyroid hormone is extracted from parathyroid glands but is too antigenic for long term use. Large doses (1–5 mg) of vitamin D are used, often with calcium supplements, to maintain the serum calcium level. Regular monitoring of plasma calcium is necessary to avoid intoxication.

(c) Prophylaxis in infants and pregnant or lactating women is usually recommended, although a normal diet contains an adequate amount of the vitamin. The children of coloured immigrants in Britain occasionally develop rickets, and it is assumed that the skin pigmentation of these patients prevents the compensatory effect of ultraviolet irradiation of the skin.

Vitamin K

Vitamin K is responsible for the production of prothrombin and clotting factors VII, IX and X. It is found in a variety of foods of animal and plant origin, and is synthesized by the normal gut flora. It is available for administration in several forms, the naturally occurring phytomenadione and the synthetic forms menaphthone, menadiol and acetomenaphthone. The synthetic derivatives can cause haemolysis in large doses.

Indications for use

(a) Reversal of anticoagulation. Coumarin and indanedione anti-coagulants inhibit the production of prothrombin and factors VII, IX and X. This can be overcome by vitamin K when haemorrhagic complications demand immediate action. Phytomenadione is the most satisfactory for this purpose.

(b) Haemorrhagic disease of the newborn. Low levels of prothrombin and factors VII, IX and X are found in the newborn because of the lack of normal intestinal flora. This is exaggerated in premature infants, and may cause haemorrhagic complications. Routine prophylactic vitamin K is given in many centres. Synthetic analogues displace bilirubin from its plasma-protein binding sites, causing kernicterus if too large a dose is given.

(c) Jaundice. Naturally-occurring vitamin K is fat soluble and requires bile for its normal absorption. Hypoprothrombinaemia accompanying obstructive jaundice responds rapidly to administration of vitamin K, but when liver disease is present the response may be poor.

(d) Intestinal disorders. Hypoprothrombinaemia can occur in steatorrhoea, and when the bacterial flora of the gut are disturbed by oral sulphonamide or broad-spectrum antibiotic treatment.

Iron

The daily requirement of iron is 1 mg in men and 2–3 mg in menstruating women. The absorption from the gut is regulated to the requirement, but although an excess of iron is contained in the average diet much of it is unavailable for absorption. Iron preparations contain ferrous salts which are readily available. Iron deficiency anaemia can occur with a poor diet, with gastrointestinal disorders, during pregnancy or in chronic blood loss. Even a good diet needs supplementing with iron salts in the treatment of established anaemia, for the body stores of about 1500 mg have been depleted.

Oral iron preparations. A number of ferrous salts can be used. Ferrous sulphate is the cheapest, and is satisfactory for most patients. Most preparations contian 50–60 mg of iron. Sometimes it produces nausea, particularly when taken on an empty stomach. In this case ferrous gluconate or fumarate may be tried. Delayed-release preparations reduce gastrointestinal symptoms, but are more expensive and the release of iron from them is less certain. Ferrous succinate is better absorbed than the other salts, and thus the dose is smaller.

Ferric ammonium citrate is available as a liquid preparation, but it can cause blackening of the teeth. Iron edetate is also available, but is expensive.

All iron preparations should be kept out of the reach of children, for they can cause serious acute poisoning.

Interactions with tetracyclines are discussed on p. 271.

Parenteral preparations. Occasionally parenteral preparations are indicated, usually because the patient is considered to be unreliable in drug taking, but sometimes because oral preparations are poorly tolerated or are not absorbed adequately because of gastrointestinal disease. The dose must be calculated from the haemoglobin level, as a large excess can produce haemochromatosis.

Two preparations are available, iron-dextran and iron-sorbitol-citrate. The first of these is the more satisfactory as iron-sorbitol-citrate is partly excreted in the urine. They are given by deep intramuscular injection. A painful local reaction occasionally occurs, and brown staining of the skin is caused by leakage back along the needle track to the subcutaneous tissues. Iron-dextrose can be given as a single replacement dose by intravenous infusion after suitable dilution, although this is seldom required in practice and is associated with a higher incidence of adverse reactions. These include fever, rashes, joint pains, nausea and headache. Anaphylactic shock occurs rarely.

18

Drugs in malignant disease

Alkylating agents

These drugs possess reactive alkyl radicals which link together opposed guanine molecules on the two strands of deoxyribonucleic acid (DNA), preventing the DNA helix uncoiling and so arresting its replication. In this way, mitosis is prevented, particularly in those tissues which show the greatest rate of cell division. In normal subjects this includes the haemopoietic system, the gastrointestinal mucosa and the skin. The faster rate of mitosis in malignant tissues provides the rationale for the use of these drugs in patients with such conditions.

Mustards. Mustine hydrochloride, the original nitrogen mustard, was noted to produce leucopenia in subjects dyiny from exposure to mustard gas in the First World War. It has to be given intravenously, and commonly produces nausea and vomiting within 1 to 4 hours after administration. Pancytopenia occurs with excessive dosage. Its main value is in Hodgkin's diease and lymphosarcoma.

Chlorambucil, a phenylbutyric acid mustard, affects primarily the lymphoid tissues and is of particular value in chronic lymphatic leukaemia, lymphosarcoma and Waldenstrom's macroglobulinaemia. It has also given good results in Hodgkin's disease, ovarian carcinoma and seminoma. Unlike mustine it can be administered orally, and is less damaging to the haemopoietic system, although with excessive dosage or prolonged therapy bone marrow depression may occur.

Melphalan, a phenylalanine mustard, is used mainly in the treatment of myelomatosis.

Cyclophosphamide, a cyclic phosphoramide mustard, is of particular value in Hodgkin's disease, myelomatosis, chronic lymphatic leukaemia and ovarian carcinoma. It produces alopecia more readily than oher alkylating agents, and irritant metabolites in the urine may produce a chemical cystitis. It may be given orally or intravenously.

245

Ifosfamide is structurally related to cyclophosphamide and may be more active against soft tissue sarcoma and some lung carcinomas. Like cyclophosphamide, it can produce a chemical cystitis, which appears to be due to an inactive metabolite acrolein. Bladder irrigation with sulphydryl (−SH) donors such as N-acetyl cysteine (see page 289) can protect the bladder mucosa against the effects of acrolein.

Lomustine (CCNU) and carmustine (BCNU) are nitrosoureas with relatively high lipid solubility, and so cross the blood-brain barrier. They are therefore used to treat brain tumours as well as other forms of malignancy. Their use is limited by severe bone marrow depression that often begins 3 to 4 weeks after treatment.

Some tumour cells possess hormone receptors, and this has been exploited with estramustine which is a stable combination of mustine with oestradiol, designed to treat tumours with oestrogen receptors, such as metastatic prostatic cancer. Prednimustine, which is chlorambucil linked to a corticosteroid, is being assessed in leukaemias and lymphomas.

Ethyleneimmonium compounds. Thiotepa, which is the only important member of this group of alkylating agents, has proved effective in some patients with malignant melanoma, and carcinoma of the breast and ovary. It may be administered orally or intravenously, and may be injected directly into a body cavity containing effusions secondary to metastatic involvement. Like other alkylating agents, prolonged therapy or excessive dosage may produce bone marrow depression.

Dimethanesulphonates. Busulphan is the most important member of this group and is of particular value in the treatment of chronic myeloid leukaemia, its action in small doses being largely restricted to the myeloid series in the bone marrow, selectively suppressing proliferation of granulocytic cells and to a lesser extent platelet production. It is administered orally, and commonly produces hyperpigmentation of the skin. A rare but important adverse effect is interstitial pulmonary fibrosis similar to that which may follow the use of hexamethonium. Treosulfan is a derivative of busulphan used to treat ovarian cancer. Its unwanted effects are similar to busulphan.

Antimetabolites

An antimetabolite closely resembles a particular metabolite in chemical structure and successfully competes with it as a substrate in an enzyme system. This results in blockade of the particular metabolic pathway involved, which in the case of drugs used in cancer chemotherapy is usually in the synthetic pathway of nucleic acids.

Folic acid antagonists. Methotrexate competes with folic acid for the enzyme folic acid reductase which is responsible for conversion of folic acid to tetrahydrofolic acid, a coenzyme in the methylation of deoxyuridylic acid to form thymidylic acid. It therefore blocks the synthesis of the latter and consequently of DNA. Its main use is by oral adminstration in the maintenance treatment of acute lymphoblastic leukaemia, and it may be administered intrathecally to control neurological complications of the disease. It is also very effective in the treatment of chorion carcinoma. When given by intra-arterial perfusion in regional chemotherapy, its systemic toxic effects can be reduced or prevented by parenteral injection of tetrahydrofolic acid. Among its toxic effects are leucopenia and thrombocytopenia, megaloblastic anaemia, alopecia, ulcerative stomatitis and hepatic necrosis and fibrosis.

Purine antagonists. 6-Mercaptopurine acts at several different points in the early stages. of purine synthesis so blocking the production of DNA. Like methotrexate, its most frequent use is in the maintenance of acute leukaemia.

Azathioprine is a derivative of 6-mercaptopurine which is used primarily as an immunosuppressant agent in patients receiving organ transplants.

Pyrimidine antagonists. Cytosine arabinoside (cytarabine) interferes with DNA synthesis by blocking the formation of deoxycytidylic acid from cytidylic acid. It is a valuable drug in the treatment of acute myeloblastic leukaemia, particularly when used in combination with other drugs such as daunorubicin. 5-Fluoruracil, like cytarabine, interferes with nucleic acid synthesis and appears to be of benefit in some patients with carcinoma of the ovary, stomach, intestinal tract and breast.

Plant and extracts

Colchicine, derived from the autumn crocus, inhibits cell division by arresting mitosis in the metaphase. Although it is not used clinically because of its toxic effects, its derivative demicolcine is sometimes used in chronic myeloid leukaemia and Hodgkin's disease.

Vinca alkaloids come from the West Indian periwinkle. Vinblastine is a valuable drug in the treatment of Hodgkin's disease and chorioncarcinoma, and vincristine is used in combination with prednisolone in the primary treatment of acute lymphoblastic leukaemia. They are administered intravenously. Like colchicine they both cause metaphase arrest. Vincristine is markedly neurotoxic, producing motor, sensory and autonomic neuropathies. Vindesine is a newer alkaloid that has shown activity in acute lymphoblastic leukaemia, lymphomas, melanoma, bronchial carcinoma and testicular teratoma. Like vincristine it is neurotoxic.

Etoposide, an alkaloid derived from podophyllotoxin is used for treating carcinoma of the lung and testicular teratoma. Adverse effects include alopecia and bone marrow suppression.

Antibiotics

Actinomycin D, formed during the growth of various *Streptomyces* species, is used in the treatment of Wilm's tumour in children and in chorioncarcinoma and rhabdomyosarcoma. It probably acts by combining with DNA, inhibiting the synthesis of RNA and protein. Daunorubicin (rubidomycin, daunomycin), also derived from certain *Streptomyces* strains, interferes with the synthesis of DNA and RNA by combining with performed DNA. It is one of the most effective drugs in the treatment of acute myeloblastic leukaemia, particularly when used in combination with cytosine arabinoside. It has marked marrow depressant and cardiotoxic properties. Streptozotocin has been successfully used in treating insulin-secreting islet-cell carcinomas of the pancreas. Bleomycin is preferentially concentrated in epithelial tissues and has been used to treat cancers of the mouth and oesophagus, as well as lymphomas. It has been used intrapleurally in patients with mesothelioma of the pleura. It may produce wide-spread lung fibrosis. Cyclosporin A is a potent immunosuppressive agent which is used in transplant surgery to suppress rejection (p. 227). Mitomycin is used to treat gastric cancer, in intermittent high doses, to reduce the risk of severe delayed bone marrow suppression.

Platinum complexes

Platinum diaminodichloride (cis-platinum) appears to inhibit DNA synthesis, and in low concentrations achieves this without significant effect on RNA or protein synthesis. It is given intravenously and distributed throughout all tissues with higher concentrations in liver and kidney. As well as producing nausea, vomiting, bone marrow suppression and immunosuppression, it can also cause renal tubular necrosis and damage to the cochlea. It appears to have a similar spectrum of therapeutic activity to the alkylating agents.

Other drugs

Procarbazine is a methylhydrazine which suppresses mitosis by prolonging interphase and causing a high percentage of chromatid breaks. It is effective in the treatment of Hodgkin's disease.

L-Asparaginase is an enzyme which breaks down the amino acid L-asparagine to aspartic acid and ammonia. It therefore reduces the body pool of asparagine on which some neoplastic cells may be dependent. It is derived from cultures of *Escherichia coli* and of *Erwinia carotovera*, and is particularly effective in inducing remissions in acute lymphatic leukaemia in children, although resistance to it rapidly develops.

Hormones

Prednisolone is effective in many malignant disorders of the reticulo-endothelial system. It suppresses activity of lymphoid tissue and may be associated with an increase in cells of the myeloid and platelet series. In addition, it may reverse the bleeding tendency and inhibit the auto-agglutination which is often found in these disorders.

Oestrogens, androgens and progestogens are used in the treatment of neoplasia in organs which are normally under the influence of the sex hormones, such as the breast, ovary, uterus and prostate.

Thyroid hormone, administered as thyroxine or desiccated thyroid extract, may cause regression of differentiated carcinoma of the thyroid and its metastases.

Radioactive compounds

Radioactive iodine (^{131}I) is concentrated in thyroid tissue and is used for the detection and treatment of inoperable thyroid carcinoma and its metastases. Only about 15% of tumours are sufficiently well differentiated to concentrate the iodine, however, and so its effectiveness is limited to relatively few patients.

Radioactive gold (^{123}Au) is used to inhibit effusions in serous cavities such as the pleura and peritoneum.

Radioactive phosphorus (^{32}P) accumulates in haemopoietic tissue, producing a reduction in red and white cell counts and it has been used, therefore, in the treatment of polycythaemia.

Cytotoxic activity and the cell cycle

There is experimental evidence from the action of cytotoxic drugs on mouse leukaemia that they may be classified according to their predominant effect on the cell cycle. Cells not actively dividing are said to be resting in the Go state. In the actively dividing cell, the mitosis or M phase is followed by the G_1 interphase; then follows the DNA synthetic or S phase; finally the G_2 interphase before the next M phase. In the mouse leukaemia model, high dose mustine acts non-specifically on dividing and resting cells. Methotrexate, cytosine arabinoside and the vinca alkaloids only kill cells in their proliferating phase and then only at certain stages of the cell cycle. Chlorambucil, cyclophosphamide, flurouracil, busulphan, and the antibiotic cytotoxic agents kill only proliferating cells, but throughout their cell cycle. *Cycle specific* drugs are those that can destroy proliferating cells throughout the generation cycle; *phase specific* drugs affect only one or more phases of the cycle. The relevance of this classification to human oncology is not yet established.

FURTHER READING

McEwen J, Slevin M L 1983 Recent advances in cancer chemotherapy. In: Turner P, Shand D G (eds) Recent advances in clinical pharmacology, Vol. 3, Churchill Livingstone, Edinburgh

19

Antimicrobial drugs

Modern antimicrobial therapy began in 1935 with the publication by Domagk of the results of a successful trial on an azo dye, Prontosil, in the treatment of erysipelas. The development of other related compounds led to the introduction of potent sulphonamides into clinical practice, and a dramatic reduction in the mortality from puerperal fever immediately followed. These compounds must be distinguished from antibiotics which, by definition, are substances produced by micro-organisms antagonistic to the growth of others in high dilution. The first antibiotic to be used in man was penicillin (in 1940), following the work of Chain and Florey on an extract of cultures of a mould, *Penicillium notatum*. Since this time many clinically-useful antibiotics have been isolated from bacteria from the most unlikely of sources, e.g. cephalosporins were first isolated from a mould grown from a sewage outfall in Sardinia.

Mode of action

It is usual to divide antibacterial drugs into those which are bactericidal, i.e. able to kill the bacteria, and those which are bacteriostatic i.e. preventing their growth, but not killing them. Subsequent destruction of bacteria following treatment with a bacteriostatic drug is brought about by natural defence reactions. This division can be important in practice, for antagonism can occur between drugs from one group and those from the other. Some drugs are bacteriostatic in low concentrations and bactericidal at higher concentrations.

Antimicrobials produce their effect by interfering with one or more vital metabolic pathways in the organism.

(*a*) *Inhibition of folic acid production.* Unlike man, bacteria synthesize their own folic acid, and this substance is essential as a co-enzyme for the normal production of nucleotides required for cell division. Sulphonamides have a structural similarity to *p*-aminobenzoic acid, which is a precursor of folic acid. The drug competes with this precursor and is preferentially incorporated into the folic acid molecule (Fig. 19.1). The resulting compound is inactive, and bacteria fail to divide.

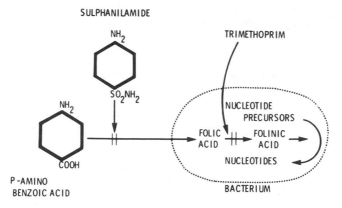

Fig. 19.1 Sites of action of sulphonamides and trimethoprim.

Trimethoprim acts at a different point in the folic acid pathway, selectively inhibiting the bacterial enzyme dihydrofolate reductase. Combination of this compound with sulphamethoxazole produces a preparation with potent antibacterial actions (co-trimoxazole).

(*b*) *Inhibition of cell wall synthetis.* The bacterial cell wall is synthesized from a variety of amino acids, nucleotides and mucopeptides, and a number of points in the complex metabolic pathway can be inhibited by antibiotics. The β-lactam bond of penicillins and cephalosporins is a structural analogue of D-alanyl-D-alanine, part of the pentapeptide of muramic acid, a major cell wall component. These antibiotics interfere with alanine transpeptidation and prevent the final stage of cross linking in the cell wall. This leads to the production of a weak cell wall, resulting in subsequent lysis of the cells (i.e. bactericidal effect). Other antibiotics, e.g. bacitracin, vancomycin and cycloserine, act at earlier stages of the pathway and have a different spectrum of activity.

(*c*) *Inhibition of protein synthesis.* Bacteria, like other cells manufacture proteins from amino acids in the cytoplasmic ribosomes. Messenger RNA specifies the sequence of amino acids for the protein being produced, and transfer RNA transfers the appropriate amino acids as they are required. Antibiotics can disturb this process in a number of ways. Chloramphenicol inhibits the transfer of the growing peptide chain to the amino acid which has been newly attached to the ribosome. Tetracyclines interfere with the linkage necessary for this transfer. Macrolides and lincomycin disturb the translocation of the messenger RNA which normally brings the next codon opposite the amino acid attachment site. Finally, streptomycin and the other aminoglycosides attach themselves to the ribosome and cause misreading of information supplied by messenger RNA, and the resulting protein contains misplaced amino acids, making it unable to fulfil its normal role.

Drug resistance

Resistance to the action of an antimicrobial drug can be one of two types, (a) drug-tolerance, in which the bacteria become capable of growing in the presence of the drug, or (b) drug-destruction, in which an enzyme is produced by the bacteria which destroys the drug, even though the organisms themselves may remain fully sensitive to the drug's action. The second of these mechanisms is responsible for resistance to penicillins and cephalosporins. Staphylococci, many coliforms and a few other organisms can produce enzymes, β-lactamases (penicillinases), which can open the β-lactam bond and destroy its activity. The older penicillins are highly susceptible, but some of the newer compounds are relatively resistant. Cephalosporins are, in general, most resistant to β-lactamases than penicillins.

The development of tolerance is explained either by the selective growth of a small number of naturally-resistant bacteria or by the occurrence of spontaneous mutation, giving rise to drug-resistant organisms. The resistant bacteria become dominant as the drug-sensitive ones are destroyed. Other factors may sometimes be involved, such as transmission of the ability to produce penicillinase from one organism to another by a bacteriophage, or transference of plasmids (extrachromosomal genetic particles) from one species to another. This latter mechanism is known to account for the frequent possession of drug-resistance by enterobacteria which have never been exposed to the drug. This is often termed 'infectious' resistance.

Principles of treatment

The object of treatment with an antimicrobial drug is to produce at the site of infection a concentration of the drug which is higher than the minimal effective concentration, and which is maintained at the level until the organisms have been eliminated. Failure to meet these requirements encourages the development of resistance. If the drug is being given for a systemic infection it is preferable to give it parenterally if there is any doubt about its absorption (e.g. penicillin).

The frequency of administration is determined by the half-life of the drug in the serum. When renal and hepatic function are normal the standard dose intervals for a particular drug can be adhered to, but sometimes it is necessary to modify them. For example, the liver of the neonate is unable to metabolise many drugs adequately during the first month or so of its life, and this accounts for the 'grey baby' syndrome which developed when premature infants were given prophylactic chloramphenicol. Aminoglycoside antibiotics are almost entirely eliminated in the urine, so that impairment of renal function will cause accumulation of the drug, with subsequent 8th nerve damage, if normal doses are given. In this instance frequent measurement of the serum concentration of the drug is essential, especially in the first few days of treatment until a plateau level has been reached. Computer programmes have been written to predict the steady-state level from the kinetics of a single dose, but tables have been published to guide the clinician who lacks this sophisticated help.

The choice of drug for a particular infection is based on (a) the clinical picture (in some infections, e.g. syphilis, the causative organism is invariably sensitive to a particular antibiotic), (b) the bacteriological diagnosis (which is more often the case, as many infections, e.g. pneumonia, can be caused by one of several organisms), and (c) in vitro sensitivity tests. With any one organism there may be a choice of several antimicrobial drugs, and guidance by sensitivity tests can be invaluable in these circumstances. It is usually necessary, however, to start treatment before bacteriological reports are available, and prediction about the type of organism and its sensitivity must be made. Factors such as the cost and potential toxicity of a drug must be taken into account when deciding between several different treatments to which the organisms are equally sensitive. A number of deaths are caused each year by sensitivity to antibiotic drugs, especially penicillins. In addition, there is a considerable morbidity, which is less easy to assess, produced by their toxic actions. It is indefensible when these reactions occur in a patient treated with a powerful drug for a trivial infection, or when the infection (e.g. a common cold) did not justify antibiotic treatment in the first place. Greater discrimination in the use of these drugs would also delay the acquisition of resistance, a problem which has grown almost as rapidly as the number of available drugs has grown.

In general, narrow-spectrum antibiotics are preferable to broad-spectrum agents which, by suppressing commensal bacteria, may encourage, superinfection with resistant organisms, particularly fungi such as *Candida albicans*.

Most infections are successfully treated with a single drug, but occasionally combined treatment is justified. This has two main purposes, (a) to increase bactericidal potency by a synergic effect, and (b) to prevent the development of bacterial resistance. These principles are exemplified by the management of tuberculosis with combinations of two or three drugs. It is acceptable to combine a bacteriostatic drug with another bacteriostat, or one bactericidal drug with another, but drugs with a different type of action should not be mixed because antagonism may occur. Bactericidal antibiotics (e.g. penicillin) produce their effect on multiplying bacteria, and the presence of a bacteriostatic drug (e.g. tetracycline) will prevent this action.

The route of administration of an antimicrobial drug depends upon its physicochemical nature and on the site of infection to be treated. Streptomycin, for example, is strongly basic and poorly absorbed, and it must therefore be given by injection for systemic infections. A related drug, neomycin, is frequently given orally, however, for bowel infections. Local infections, e.g. conjunctivitis, can be treated by local administration of drugs, but allergy can result from repeated use, particularly of penicillins. Abscesses, e.g. a tuberculous abscess in the lung or empyema, may be walled-off with fibrous tissue which is poorly penetrated by antibiotics, and may have to be treated surgically or by local injection of the drug.

When antibiotics are given in combination the two drugs should not be mixed in the same syringe unless it is known that they are compatible. Precipitation of one drug by a change in pH is a particular hazard. Similarly, a drug given by intravenous infusion should never be added to blood or amino acid solutions. They should be given separately in dextrose or saline, as the manufacturers recommend.

Synthetic antimicrobials

Sulphonamides

The development of the sulphonamides has produced, in addition to a large number of antibacterial compounds, several clinically useful antidiabetic drugs and a carbonic anhydrase inhibitor with diuretic and anticonvulsant properties (acetazolamide). Those with antimicrobial actions have a wide spectrum of activity covering both Gram-positive and Gram-negative bacteria, with a few exceptions. Strepococci (except *Strep. faecalis*), pneumococci, gonococci and meningococci are highly sensitive, although resistance was acquired early by some species when sulphonamides were widely used, especially gonococci. Resistant meningococci have only recently been reported. Sulphonamides now have a rather restricted use, but remain valuable drugs in urinary tract infections, meningococcal meningitis and bowel infections. The development of resistance is the result of a mutation which produces a folic acid synthetase less sensitive to the action of the drug.

Since the introduction of these compounds the aims of further development have been to produce more potent antibacterial derivatives, which reached a peak with the synthesis of sulphathiazole and sulphadiazine, and to produce compounds whose pharmacokinetics suited them to specific uses. For example, some drugs are rapidly absorbed and rapidly excreted in the urine, sometimes by tubular secretion, making them suitable for use as urinary antiseptics. Other compounds are more slowly excreted and maintain a therapeutic serum level for much longer after a single dose. This property makes them more suitable for the treatment of systemic infections as the antibacterial effect is more constant despite longer dose intervals. Some drugs are slightly absorbed, if at all, and are suitable for treating bowel infections. These differences are summarized in Table 19.1.

Sulphonamides are conjugated in the liver to form acetyl derivates, which are excreted in the urine. They lack antibacterial actions. The proportions of parent compound to acetyl-derivative in the urine varies from one drug to another, and this is important in determining potency in urinary infections. The solubility of drug or metabolite in urine is low with some drugs, especially sulphathiazole and sulphadiazine. This can lead to crystal formation in the renal tubules, causing haematuria and blockage of tubules or ureter. This problem is minimized by giving alkali with the drug, as solubility is increased in an alkaline urine.

Acetylation of sulphadimidine, like that of isoniazid, is bimodally distributed, i.e. some subjects are slow acetylators, and others are fast. As there is correspondence between the rate of acetylation of these two drugs, sulphadimidine has been used to identify slow acetylators before starting isoniazid therapy.

Table 19.1

	Short acting	Medium acting	Long acting	Non-absorbed
Absorption	Good	Good	Good	v. poor
Distribution	Wide	Wide	Wide	—
Half-life	<6 hours	Up to 20 hours	Up to 40 hours	—
Excretion	Rapid	Moderate	Slow	—
Frequency of administration	4–6 hourly	12 hourly	Once daily	—
Uses	Systemic infections Urinary infections Eye infections	Systemic infections	Systemic infections	Bowel infections
Examples	Sulphadimidine Sulphafurazole Sulphathiazole Sulphamethizole Sulphacetamide (eye drops only)	Sulphamethoxazole Sulphadiazine	Sulphamethoxypyridazine Sulphadimethoxine[a]	Phthalysulphathiazole Sulphasalazine[b]

[a] A single dose gives a therapeutic serum level for a week.
[b] Compound of sulphapyridine and salicyclic acid, used in ulcerative colitis.

Sulphonamides are bound to plasma proteins to a variable extent, the most highly bound being sulphamethizole and sulphamethoxy-pyridazine, which are over 90% bound. This explains the occurrence of kernicterus of newborn whose mothers have received sulphonamide drugs shortly before delivery. Displacement of bilirubin from its binding sites leads to excessive transfer across the poorly formed blood-brain barrier, and staining of the basal ganglia (kernicterus) occurs, causing a disturbance of their function.

In addition to the adverse effects already mentioned, sulphonamides can produce hypersensitivity reactions, including skin rashes, polyarteritis and the Stevens-Johnson syndrome. Leukopenia occasionally occurs, and haemolytic anaemia from production of methaemoglobin is seen in patients who have a deficiency of glucose-6-phosphate dehydrogenase in their erythrocytes.

Trimethoprim

Trimethoprim has a strongly synergic effect with sulphonamides (Fig. 19.1) and a combination of trimethoprim with sulphamethoxazole was first introduced as a broad spectrum antibacterial preparation in 1969. Sulphamethoxazole was chosen for the combination as it has a serum half-life similar to that of trimethoprim. The combination has the official name co-trimoxazole, and contains one part of trimethoprim to five parts of the sulphonamide. This proportion produces serum levels of approximately 1:20 in favour of the sulphonamide, and this ratio is optimum for antibacterial effect against most species. However, concentration ratios in tissues vary enormously, and may not be optimum for an antibacterial effect.

Whereas trimethoprim and the sulphonamide drug are bacteriostatic when given alone, the combination may be bactericidal. In theory, the spectrum of activity of the combination is wider than that of the constituent drugs alone, and it has been widely used in infections where a broad-spectrum antibiotic is indicated, e.g. mixed respiratory and urinary tract infections. In practice, however, co-trimoxazole has a proven advantage only in gonorrhoea and *Bacteriodes fragilis* infections. In urinary tract and respiratory infections trimethoprim is being used alone increasingly. Trimethoprim is largely excreted unchanged in the urine.

Adverse effects have been comparatively few, although nausea was common when higher doses were being used in early trials. Although mammalian dihydrofolate reductase is 50 000 times less sensitive to trimethoprim than is its bacterial counterpart, long-term co-trimoxazole therapy can produce neutropenia, thrombocytopenia and even aplastic anaemia. Folate-deficient patients with megaloblastic changes are particularly sensitive. Large doses have caused teratogenic effects in rats, and therefore its use cannot be commended during pregnancy. When renal function is impaired, the sulphonamide component accumulates more than trimethoprim and may cause toxicity.

Co-trifamole is a combination of sulphamoxole and trimethoprim, and has a similar spectrum of activity to co-trimoxazole.

Urinary antiseptics

A number of compounds are active against the common urinary pathogens, are excreted in high concentration in the urine and because of their rapid excretion, have little systemic antibacterial effect. These drugs are labelled 'urinary antiseptics'.

Hexamine mandelate. This is a compound of hexamine and mandelic acid. The former liberates formaldehyde in an acid medium, and this substance is inhibitory to all species of bacterium. To be effective the pH of the urine should be kept below 5.5, which is not easy to do in practice. Mandelic acid is combined with hexamine with this aim in mind, for it is excreted unchanged and is itself inhibitory to bacteria. However, it is seldom adequate to maintain urinary acidity without the addition of other acidifying agents such as ammonium chloride, ascorbic acid or methionine. The latter agent increases the output of urinary sulphates, but by its effect on trans-sulphuration reactions it can cause vitamin B_6 deficiency. Hexamine will release formaldehyde in the stomach and therefore has to be enteric-coated.

Urine infected with urea-splitting organisms, e.g. *Proteus*, cannot effectively be acidified, and it may be necessary to use a drug which is active in an alkaline urine, such as an aminoglycoside antibiotic.

Nitrofurantoin. This drug is particularly effective in *Esch. coli* infections, but is not active against *Pseudomonas* or some *Proteus* strains. It is most effective in an acid urine, into which it is rapidly excreted and to which it imparts a fluorescent yellow colour. Only about one third of the oral dose can be recovered from the urine, the remainder being broken down in the tissues. Adequate antibacterial levels are reached in the kidney interstitium and the drug can be used for treating acute pyelonephritis.

Adverse effects include gastrointestinal upsets, allergic reactions and peripheral eosinophilia. Peripheral neuropathy, not responsive to vitamin B therapy, occurs with prolonged or excessive therapy, particularly in the presence of impaired renal function, but is usually reversible. Renal function should be investigated before prescribing a prolonged course. Haemolytic anaemia has been reported in patients with glucose-6-phosphate dehydrogenase deficiency.

Nalidixic acid. The spectrum of activity of this compound is similar to that of nitrofurantoin. It is rapidly excreted in the urine mainly as metabolites, some of which are inactive. Resistance readily occurs, lessening its usefulness for treating chronic infections or for long-term suppressive therapy. Raised intracranial pressure has accompanied its use in children.

Cinoxacin is chemically related to nalidixic acid and has the advantage that it needs to be given only twice daily rather than four times daily.

Metronidazole

This synthetic compound has been used for some years in trichomonal vaginitis, and in *Entamoeba histolytica* and *Giardia lamblia* infections of the alimentary tract. More recently, its high activity against anaerobic bacteria such as *Bacteriodes fragilis* has been recognised and it has become a mainstay in the treatment of localized and systemic infections caused by these organisms, and for prophylaxis in elective colonic surgery. It can be administered orally, intravenously or by rectal suppository for systemic therapy and its excellent absorption from the latter route has made parenteral administration, which is expensive, generally unnecessary. Vaginal pessaries can be used for local trichomonal infections, but systemic absorption from this site also is good.

Metronidazole diffuses well into tissue and body fluids including abscess cavities and the central nervous system. It is partly metabolized to inactive products, and partly excreted unchanged. Its plasma half-life is 8–10 hours in patients with normal hepatic and renal function. Adverse effects include central nervous system toxicity (vertigo, ataxia, seizures), peripheral neuropathy, nausea, and vomiting, metallic taste, anorexia, diarrhoea, rashes and a disulfiram-like flushing (disulfiram is a drug which blocks alcohol metabolism at the stage of acetaldehyde formation, and is used in treating alcoholism). Although it is active against *Clostridium difficile*, it can also cause colitis induced by this organism (as can lincomycin and clindamycin, which are also used in treating anaerobic infections).

Tinidazole is similar in spectrum of activity, but has a longer plasma half-life and therefore requires less frequent administration.

Synthetic drugs for tuberculosis

Prolonged treatment with antimicrobial drugs is necessary to establish a cure in tuberculosis. Because the organisms readily acquire resistance to a single agent, combinations of drugs are used. The British Thoracic Association has recommended nine months chemotherapy with rifampicin plus isoniazid, with ethambutol added for the first two months, as the preferred treatment of pulmonary tuberculosis in Britain. Streptomycin can be used in place of ethambutol. Addition of pyrazinamide produces a powerful antibacterial effect in infections with resistant organisms. The antibiotics capreomycin and cycloserine are also used in resistant tuberculous infections. Only the synthetic drugs are considered here.

Isoniazid. Isonicotinic acid hydrazide (INAH) has been successfully used in treating tuberculosis since 1952. It combines high potency, cheapness (an important factor in developing countries) and low toxicity. Taken orally it is well absorbed and penetrates effectively into tissues and the cerebrospinal fluid. About 45% of Caucasians are slow inactivators (by hepatic acetylation), and this trait is genetically determined, probably by a recessive gene (p. 19). Adverse effects are confined mainly to this group, but high dosage over a prolonged period is necessary to produce these effects. Peripheral neuropathy, responding to pyridoxine treatment, is the most serious. Pyridoxine should be given prophylactically when high doses are administered. Other adverse effects, such as restlessness, insomnia, muscle twitching and difficulty in starting micturition also occur.

Ethambutol. This is a powerful drug without cross-resistance. It is well absorbed orally and about half the dose is excreted unchanged in the urine. In renal insufficiency a reduction in dose is necessary. In general it is well tolerated but it is toxic to the optic nerve, producing either central or periaxial retrobulbar neuritis. Evidence of decreased visual acuity or red-green colour discrimination should be sought at regular ophthalmological assessment. Peripheral neuritis may also occur.

Thioacetazone. As a cheap alternative to para-aminosalicylic acid (PAS), this drug has become popular in developing countries. It is as effective as PAS, and can be given with isoniazid as a single daily dose. It produces adverse effects more frequently, particularly in doses of about 150 mg/day.

Ethionamide. Like isoniazid, this compound is a derivative of nicotinic acid, although cross-resistance with isoniazid is not shown. It is a potent bactericide, but has a high incidence of adverse effects, particularly on the gastrointestinal tract. Prothionamide is similar, although less toxic. These drugs are useful when resistance has been acquired by the organisms to the standard drugs.

Pyrazinamide. This is another nicotinic acid derivative of moderate potency. Hepatotoxicity is the chief risk, and serum transaminase enzymes should be estimated frequently during its administration.

Antibiotics

Penicillins

No satisfactory method has been developed of synthesizing the penicillin nucleus (6-aminopenicillanic acid) for commercial production. It is obtained by large-scale culture of a high yielding strain of *Penicillium*. Phenylacetic acid is added to the medium in order to encourage the production of benzyl side chains, giving benzyl penicillin (penicillin G). This side chain can be removed enzymatically for the manufacture of newer semi-synthetic penicillins with alternative side chains.

Benzyl penicillin. As the potassium salt this is known as 'soluble' or 'crystalline' penicillin. It is highly soluble but is unstable at acid pH, and for this reason is poorly active by mouth. After intramuscular injection it is rapidly absorbed. It diffuses well into the tissues but is not found in very high concentration in the CSF. In meningitis the concentration rises higher, owing to fluid exudation, but intrathecal injection is often used to supplement the levels, even though distribution throughout the CSF is incomplete.

Urinary excretion of benzyl penicillin is extremely rapid, being largely by tubular secretion. In order to maintain an effective serum level large doses have to be given at frequent intervals. In early clinical trials this severely hampered treatment as only small amounts of penicillin were available, and the drug had to be re-extracted from the patient's urine. Tubular secretion can be inhibited by concurrent administration of probenecid, and this will produce higher serum levels for the same dose. In practice this is seldom necessary except in some cases of streptococcal endocarditis.

An alternative method of prolonging the duration of action has been employed in preparations whose absorption from the site of injection is delayed. Procaine penicillin, an equimolar compound of penicillin and procaine, is administered as a suspension of crystals which have low solubility. Effective levels can be maintained by a single daily injection. Benethamine penicillin and benzathine penicillin are even less soluble and produce a low concentration in the serum for 4–5 days and several weeks respectively. It is important to bear in mind, however, that the serum level achieved is determined by a dynamic equilibrium between rate of absorption and rate of excretion, and as the latter is unchanged the levels are inevitably considerably lower with long-acting preparations. This makes them unsuitable for acute infections.

Benzyl penicillin is active against most Gram-positive and some Gram-negative organisms, but the latter tend to be less sensitive. Haemolytic streptococci and pneumococci are always highly sensitive and because it has a powerfully bactericidal action, benzyl penicillin remains the drug of choice in these infections. Staphylococci and gonococci are also highly sensitive but resistant strains have become so widespread that alternative drugs are usually preferable unless the results of in vitro sensitivity tests are to hand. Resistance is usually the result of penicillinase production by the bacteria, and this may interfere also with the effect of the drug on other organisms present at the site of the infection which are intrinsically sensitive to the drug. Benzyl penicillin is to be preferred for treating meningococcal infections, for the organism is now often resistant to sulphonamides. Benzyl penicillin for a longer-acting preparation are still the treatment of choice for syphilis.

Benzyl penicillin has three main disadvantages, (a) it is destroyed by gastric acid, (b) it is inactivated by penicillinase and (c) its spectrum of activity is too restricted. Efforts to overcome these defects have been successful.

Acid-resistant penicillins. There are two acid-resistant penicillins in common use for oral administration: phenoxymethyl penicillin (penicillin V) and phenoxyethyl penicillin (phenethicillin).

The first of these is produced by the addition of phenoxyacetic acid to the culture medium, whereas the second is semi-synthetic. Although phenethicillin is better absorbed it is also more highly protein-bound, and the serum level of free drug differs little between the two. They are excreted rapidly and should therefore be given 4–6 hourly. Gram-negative organisms are less sensitive to these penicillins than to benzyl penicillin.

Penicillinase-resistant penicillins. These penicillins are semi-synthetic, and have side chains which protect the β-lactam ring of the penicillin nucleus from the actions of penicillinase (β-lactamase). However, they are much less active than benzyl penicillin against bacterial species which do not produce penicillinase.

Flucloxacillin is the most satisfactory of these for it is acid-resistant and is therefore active orally. Its absorption is better than that of cloxacillin, which must be given by intramuscular injection in the initial treatment of an acute infection. Both drugs are extensively protein-bound in the serum, which reduces their effectiveness.

Methicillin, the first penicillinase-resistant drug to be discovered, is less satisfactory. It must be injected as it is not acid-resistant, and it is much less active than cloxacillin against *Staph. aureus* and group A haemolytic streptococci. It is rapidly excreted in the urine and injections must be given every 4–6 hours. It is less protein-bound than cloxacillin.

Broad-spectrum penicillins. Ampicillin, a semi-synthetic drug with an α-aminobenzyl side chain, has almost as much activity against Gram-positive organisms as benzyl pencillin, but much greater activity against Gram-negative, particularly *H. influenzae, Proteus mirabilis, Esch. coli* and pathogenic enterobacteria. It is not penicillinase-resistant, but it is acid-resistant and although not very well absorbed, it gives satisfactory plasma levels when administered orally. It is of particular use in urinary infections and mixed respiratory infections but it should not be used in streptococcal pharyngitis in which simple penicillins are as effective, less expensive and less likely to produce a skin rash. As it is active against meningococci, pneumococci and *H. influenzae* it is valuable in meningitis, particularly when the organism cannot be isolated. However, resistance to the latter organism has been reported, and therefore chloramphenicol might be a better choice in life-threatening *Haemophilus* infections. Although excreted largely in the urine, its concentration in bile is high and this makes it suitable for treating typhoid carrier state. Amoxycillin is similar to ampicillin, but is better absorbed, and is therefore given in lower dosage. Pivampicillin, bacampicillin and talampicillin are esters of ampicillin which are hydrolysed in the intestinal mucosa and portal system to the parent compound. They are also better absorbed. They cannot, however, be given parenterally as the unhydrolysed compound may be toxic.

Antipseudomonal penicillins. These have much the same spectrum activity as ampicillin but are also active against *Pseudomonas aeruginosa*, an organism against which the earlier antibiotics were poorly effective. *Proteus* species and some strains of enterobacter are also susceptible. The original antipseudomonal drug, carbenicillin, has been largely superceded by ticarcillin and by three compounds known as ureidopenicillins, mezlocillin, azlocillin and piperacillin. There is little to choose between the ureidopenicillins but in general they are more active than ticarcillin against other Gram-negative organisms and against faecal streptococci. They are all given parenterally, have short half-lives of about one hour and are largely excreted by the kidneys. Carfecillin is a pro-drug of carbenicillin; it is orally absorbed and is hydrolysed into the latter. It is suitable only for pseudomonal urinary tract infections because its plasma concentration is too low for systemic infections.

Other penicillins. Mecillinam is an amidino-penicillin, having the side chain joined to the β-lactam ring by a β-amidino group. It acts only on one enzyme of the bacterial cell wall. It has a novel spectrum of activity in being particularly effective against Gram negative rods, e.g. *E. coli*, *Klebsiella* species, *Enterobacter* species, *Salmonellae* and some *Proteus* species. However, *Pseudomonas aeruginosa* and *Haemophilus influenzae* are resistant. It is inactive against Gram positive organisms. It should be reserved for treatment of resistant Gram negative urinary tract infections. Pivmecillinam is an ester of mecillinam which is hydrolysed on absorption to release mecillinam.

Adverse effects from penicillins. Benzyl penicillin is remarkably non-toxic. The only dose-related adverse effects to be reported on systemic administration are convulsions, nephritis and haemolytic anaemia, but they have only occurred with huge doses given for a long time, or in the presence of renal disease. In contrast, intrathecal administration of doses greater than 20 000 units i.e. one hundredth of the systemic dose readily produces convulsions.

Allergic reactions to all penicillins are common, particularly skin rashes. Essentially they can be divided into two types, (a) immediate anaphylactic reactions, probably produced mainly by penicillin breakdown products in the preparation, and (b) delayed serum sickness type of responses, probably caused by hapten formation by the penicilloyl derivative of penicillanic acid.

Immediate anaphylactic reactions occur in one in 10 000 to one in 100 000 patients. Although this is rare, it cannot be ignored for penicillins are widely administered, often unnecessarily, and it is a disaster when a fatal reaction occurs in a young person. It is important to inquire routinely about any previous adverse effects to penicillin before administering it to a patient.

Ampicillin rashes occur very frequently, usually appearing several days after starting treatment, or even after stopping it, and have a characteristic erythematous or maculopapular appearance. They occur in almost every patient who has infectious mononucleosis and who receives ampicillin for the accompanying sore throat. Ampicillin rashes do not necessarily indicate allergy to penicillins in general.

Local application of penicillins, e.g. eye drops, readily produces sensitization. This probably does not apply to penicillin chewing-gum, which has been popular for treating sore throats. Contact dermatitis in nurses who handle penicillins can be a problem.

Broad-spectrum penicillins taken orally frequently produce diarrhoea by altering the bowel flora.

β-lactamase inhibitors

Although some pathogens are intrinsically susceptible to penicillins, they protect themselves by producing β-lactamase. Clavulanic acid is a compound which inhibits the activity of this enzyme although itself lacking antibacterial activity. When combined with amoxycillin (as Augmentin) it extends the range of the latter compound to include *Staph. aureus*, *H. influenzae*, *N. gonorrhoea E. coli*, klebsiella and *B. fragilis*. The plasma half-life of clavulanic acid is similar to that of amoxycillin.

Cephalosporins

The nucleus of the cephalosporin molecule, 7-aminocephalosporanic acid, has a similar structure to the nucleus of the penicillins, but it differs particularly in having a higher degree of resistance to staphylococcal penicillinase. The original substance, cephalosporin C, had only moderate antibacterial activity, but side chain substitution has improved this.

The compounds developed mostly have a wide spectrum of activity against Gram-negative bacteria, including the common pathogens such as *E. coli*, *Klebsiella* species and *Proteus* species.

Except for some of the newest compounds, they are not active against *Pseudomonas aeruginosa* or faecal streptococci. Cephalosporins have found a useful place in the treatment of severe undiagnosed sepsis and resistant gonorrhoea, urinary tract and chest infections, but despite the plethora of compounds available there are few absolute indications for their use. About 10% of penicillin-allergic patients will also show allergy to cephalosporins and therefore the latter should be avoided if possible in patients who have previously reacted to a penicillin derivative.

The cephalosporins are often divided into 'generations'. The earliest compounds required parenteral administration, had only moderate resistance to β-lactamase and had a limited spectrum of activity. Some of the newer compounds can be given orally while others have an extended spectrum (i.e. including *Pseudomonas aeruginosa*) and most have a greater resistance to degradation by β-lactamase. Essentially, they can be divided into three groups, the oral agents, the earlier compounds requiring parenteral administration, and the newer extended range compounds also requiring parenteral administration.

Oral agents. These include cephalexin, cefaclor, cefadroxil and cephradine (the latter can also be given parenterally). Most *E. coli*, *Klebsiella*, *Proteus mirabilis*, *Staph. aureus*, and *N. gonorrhoeæ* are susceptible but faecal streptococci, *Enterobacter*, *Ps. aeruginosa* and *B. fragilis* are resistant. Oral absorption is good but they have short plasma half-lives and therefore require administration 3–4 times daily.

Earlier parenteral agents. Cephalothin was the first cephalosporin to be used clinically and has particularly good activity against staphylococci. Some Gram-negative bacteria are capable of producing a β-lactamase which can hydrolyse the compound. Cephaloridine has a wide spectrum of activity but is now little used because of its nephrotoxicity, which is potentiated by loop diuretics such as frusemide and ethacrynic acid. Cefuroxime and cefoxitin are particularly stable to β-lactamases and the latter compound is a drug of choice in *B. fragilis* infections, but in most other situations where a cephalosporin is indicated, cefuroxime is the most satisfactory drug in this class. These earlier parenteral agents also have short plasma half-lives.

Extended-spectrum parenteral agents. Some of the newer compounds are particularly resistant to β-lactamase hydrolysis and have good activity against enterobacteria, although at the expense of activity against Gram-positive organisms such as *Staph. aureus*. Cefotaxime and latamoxef are most useful in this respect. Cefsoludin has little activity against bacteria other than *Ps. aeruginosa* and infections with this latter organism are the only indication for its use. Some of the newer drugs have longer plasma half-lives than their earlier counterparts and twice daily administration may be possible.

Aminoglycosides

A number of antibiotics have been isolated from various strains of *Streptomyces* which are found in soil. Only a few of these are clinically useful, and their value is limited by toxic effects on the eighth cranial nerve and kidney.

Streptomycin was discovered shortly after penicillin was introduced into clinical medicine, and immediately became an important drug because of its activity against the tubercle bacillus. The aminoglycosides are active against many Gram-negative organisms but less active against Gram-positive.

Aminoglycosides are poorly absorbed and are therefore given parenterally. They are eliminated almost entirely by urinary excretion and will accumulate if renal function is impaired. This is of vital importance in elderly patients, in whom ototoxic effects are much more common unless allowance is made for reduced glomerular filtration. Urine concentrations are high and they have a powerful bactericidal effect in Gram-negative urinary infections, especially when the urine is made alkaline. When renal function is normal effective plasma concentrations are maintained for 8 hours, and therefore they should be given at 8 hourly intervals for acute infections. Plasma level monitoring is mandatory in order to minimize the risk of ototoxicity and nephrotoxicity. Blood samples are usually taken one hour after intramuscular injection (20 minutes after intravenous injection) and again immediately before the next dose. When renal function is impaired, the size and frequency of maintenance doses are determined by the plasma levels measured.

Once a mainstay of antituberculous chemotherapy, streptomycin is now little used. Bacteria can rapidly acquire resistance to it, but this can be prevented by combining it with other antibacterial drugs, such as ethambutol and INAH in tuberculosis (p. 261). It is sometimes combined with penicillin for treatment of enterococcal endocarditis. It is effective in plague, tularaemia and brucellosis. The ototoxicity of the drug is directed mainly towards the vestibular branch of the eighth nerve.

The most widely used aminoglycoside for systemic administration is gentamicin. It has much greater antibacterial activity than streptomycin; it has a broad spectrum but is inactive against the tubercle bacillus and anaerobes, and has poor activity against haemolytic streptococci and pneumococci. It is used mainly for the treatment of Gram-negative septicaemia. When it is used for the 'blind' treatment of serious microbiologically-undiagnosed septicaemia, it is usually given with a β-lactam antibiotic or metronidazole or both. In pseudomonal infections, tobramycin is preferable, and is often combined with antipseudomonal pencillin such as ticarcillin or azlocillin. Both gentamicin and tobramycin are ototoxic and nephrotoxic. Netilmicin is similar in spectrum of activity to these two drugs, but is less toxic.

Neomycin has a spectrum similar to that of streptomycin, but is more active against staphylococci and *Proteus*. It is not used systemically because it is highly toxic to the auditory branch of the eighth nerve, as well as being nephrotoxic. Resistance is acquired less readily to neomycin than to streptomycin. It has been used for the local treatment of infections, and is a constituent of many skin ointments, nasal sprays, and eye ointments but its value following topical application is doubtful. Like the other aminoglycosides, it is little absorbed when given orally and is widely used for suppression of bowel flora pre-operatively and in the prevention of hepatic coma. Its indiscriminate use leads to bacterial resistance and a prolongation of the carrier state. Although it is poorly absorbed, ototoxicity has been reported in patients with poor renal function who have received drugs orally or topically (e.g. following extensive burns).

Framycetin and paromomycin are alternatives for local application, being too toxic for systemic use.

Kanamycin has a spectrum of activity similar to that of neomycin, but is less ototoxic. It is used systemically for treating tuberculosis in which the bacilli are resistant to standard drugs. It has been replaced by gentamicin in Gram-negative septicaemia. Amikacin is a semi-synthetic derivative of kanamycin, and has an advantage over gentamicin and tobramycin in that it is active against many organisms that are resistant to the latter drugs. It should be used only in the treatment of serious gentamicin-resistant Gram-negative infections.

The ototoxicity and nephrotoxicity of aminoglycosides is potentiated by frusemide and ethacrynic acid.

Chloramphenicol

This compound was originally isolated from a strain of *Streptomyces*, but is now produced synthetically. Its introduction provided one of the first broad spectrum antibiotics which could be administered orally. Its effects are bacteriostatic rather than bactericidal, even in high concentrations. Although it has a wide spectrum of activity it is less effective against Gram-positive organisms than many other antibiotics. Its activity against Gram-negative species, however, makes it a drug of choice in certain situations, but the risk of aplastic anaemia, admittedly small, must be weighed against its potential advantages. The Committee on Safety of Medicines has recommended that it should be used only for treating typhoid fever, *H. influenzae* meningitis, and other infections where no other antibiotic will suffice. In the opinion of many clinicians chloramphenicol still has an important place in treating severe exacerbations of chronic bronchitis or severe pertussis, but its use can seldom be justified in other situations.

Bacterial resistance to chloramphenicol occurs slowly, but is seldom troublesome in countries where it is not widely used. Resistance can be of 'infectious' type among enterobacteria.

Chloramphenicol is well absorbed orally, is largely conjugated in the liver and is excreted mainly as inactive glucuronides in the urine. It diffuses particularly well into the CSF. The capacity to conjugate the drug is inadequate in the first month of life and the accumulation of the parent compound causes the 'grey-baby syndrome' in neonates and premature babies, which is characterized by vasomotor collapse.

Chloramphenicol is toxic to the bone marrow in two ways. First, it causes a dose-related depression that depends upon the inhibition of mitochondrial protein synthesis and which is entirely reversible on withdrawal. The red cell series is primarily involved. This type of toxicity occurs commonly when the dose exceeds 2 g daily for more than 10 days, but it can be predicted by regular blood counts. The second type of toxic effect is a more serious aplasia which is frequently irreversible and ultimately fatal. It is not dose related and probably results from depression of DNA synthesis is stem cells. It is rare (one in 20 000 administrations) and cannot be predicted by regular blood counts.

Chloramphenicol inhibits the metabolism of tolbutamide, oral anticoagulants and phenytoin.

Tetracyclines

The first of these compounds, chlortetracycline, was introduced in 1948, at the same time as chloramphenicol. It is obtained from a species of *Steptomyces*, and minor changes in its molecule produces two other widely used compounds, tetracycline and oxytetracycline. The spectrum of activity is similar for each of these compounds and there are only minor differences in their pharmacokinetics.

Like chloramphenicol they are active against a wide variety of organisms, including some viruses and chlamydia. They are bacteriostatic rather than bactericidal, and should not be combined with bactericidal antibiotics such as penicillin. They differ in having useful activity in a number of less common infections, such as brucellosis, tularaemia, leptospirosis, cholera, anthrax, gas gangrene, typhus, Q fever, trachoma, psittacosis, lymphogranuloma venereum and actinomycosis.

They are most commonly prescribed for chronic bronchitis. Acute upper respiratory tract infections and pneumonias should not be treated with tetracycline because many Gram-positive organisms have developed resistance. This is true also of many enterobacteria, in which resistance of the 'infectious' type may occur. Although the use of a broad-spectrum drug in mixed infections seems attractive, the widespread prescription of them for any bacteriologically-undiagnosed infection is causing an increasing problem of resistance, which may eventually severely limit their usefulness.

Tetracylines are slowly and incompletely absorbed, particularly when calcium- or iron-containing preparations are given concurrently, when chelation occurs in the bowel. They are excreted mainly into the urine, but the concentration in bile is moderately high and this prolongs their action by 'enterohepatic' circulation.

Incomplete absorption is responsible for the most troublesome of adverse effects, diarrhoea. This is very common and is probably caused mainly by elimination of normal bowel flora, allowing overgrowth of resistant staphylococci and abnormal enterobacteria. *Candida albicans* can also colonize the bowel, but addition of nystatin to tetracycline preparations does not reduce the incidence of diarrhoea and therefore there is no indication for administering these expensive preparations.

Children under the age of 8 years should not be given tetracyclines, for they are deposited in bones and teeth, producing a yellowing of the second dentition. Tetracyclines should also be avoided in pregnancy. Dose-dependent hepatocellular damage can be produced by parenteral administration.

Tetracyclines should not be used in patients known to have renal insufficiency because they accumulate, promote protein breakdown and exacerbate renal failure.

A number of newer tetracyclines have been introduced since the original three were developed, but the advantages they offer are few. Demeclocycline and methacycline have a slightly higher antibacterial activity, are excreted more slowly and therefore can be given 12 hourly rather than 6 hourly. Doxycycline is even more slowly excreted and can be given once daily. Lymecycline, minocycline and clomocycline may be better absorbed and may produce less diarrhoea. Doxycycline and minocycline do not exacerbate renal failure.

Macrolides

Erythromycin possesses a spectrum of activity similar to that of penicillin, and has been used chiefly as a substitute for this drug when sensitivity to it occurs. It is bactericidal only in higher concentrations. Bacterial resistance can become a problem, particularly with staphylococci, and addition of a second drug, such as novobiocin, is judicious if this is to be avoided. Combination with penicillin has proved useful for treating *Strep. viridans* endocarditis. It is an antibiotic of first choice in legionnaire's disease, chlamydial pneumonia, whooping cough and campylobacter enteritis.

It is moderately well absorbed and can be given as the base, stearate or estolate. The latter is better absorbed and produces higher blood levels than the base, which is not stable to gastric acid. It is excreted in high concentration in the bile and recirculates through the liver. Most of it appears to be broken down in the body, for little can be recovered from the urine.

Diarrhoea is one of the commonest adverse effects, produced by alteration in bowel flora. The estolate can produce dose-independent cholestatic jaundice.

Peptide antibiotics

These antibiotics are produced primarily by certain strains of bacilli, and comprise a polypeptide chain linked to some other group, e.g. a long chain fatty acid as in the polymyxins.

Bacitracin was first discovered in a culture from an infected wound of a child, Margaret Tracey, after whom the drug was named. It is now rarely used systemically as it is nephrotoxic and other antibiotics are more satisfactory alternatives. It is active mainly on Gram-positive cocci, particularly haemolytic streptococci of group A. It is not absorbed orally and therefore has to be injected for systemic use. It is slowly excreted in the urine, and causes degeneration of the epithelial lining of the convoluted tubules, which can lead to anuria if the drug is continued.

Bacitracin is used mainly for treating infections of the skin, and for this purpose it is often combined with neomycin and polymyxin. It has also been used for preparation of the bowel before surgery.

Polymyxins used in clinical practice are of two types, B and E. The latter was introduced as colistin. Both these compounds are bactericidal primarily against Gram-negative organisms, including many enterobacteria and, most important, *Ps. aeruginosa*. Their main use has been in infections with this latter organism, although this position is now being challenged by newer drugs, particularly gentamicin. They are not absorbed from the gut, and must be given by injection either as the sulphate of sulphomethyl derivatives. The latter are the most popular for they do not cause pain at the site of injection, as do the sulphates, and they produce fewer adverse effects.

Renal tubular damage occurs much less frequently than with bacitracin, and then usually only when there is pre-existing renal damage. Polymyxin E is less nephrotic than B. Numbness and paraesthesiae, particularly of the face, can occur, usually with the sulphates.

As with bacitracin, the polymyxins are used widely for local application to the skin, eyes and ears.

Antibiotics for penicillin-resistant organisms

One of the chief problems which has faced the bacteriologist and clinician ever since the introduction of penicillin is that of resistance, either by production of penicillinase or by mutation yielding a drug-tolerant variant. Staphylococci are notorious in this respect, and many of the antibiotics which have been developed in recent years have been aimed at these organisms. The following drugs are examples of these. They are not used widely, as the newer penicillinase-resistant penicillins and cephalosporins are currently favoured in this situation.

Fusidic acid is unusual in having a steroid structure. It is well absorbed orally as the sodium salt. Natural resistance is rare, but it can develop during treatment. For this reason it is preferable to combine it with penicillin, erythromycin or novobiocin.

Novobiocin was one of the earliest developments against resistant staphylococci and is usually given with erythromycin to delay bacterial resistance, which develops rapidly when it is used alone. It is well absorbed orally, is excreted in high concentration in the bile, and recirculates. Urticarial rashes are particularly common if it is used for more than a week.

Clindamycin, although chemically different from erythromycin, resembles it in its spectrum of activity and shows cross-resistance with it. It is more active and better absorbed than its predecessor, lincomycin. It reaches adequate concentrations in bone and has been used successfully in osteomyelitis. Its major adverse effect is pseudo-membranous colitis and its use should therefore be restricted to staphylococcal bone and joint disease and intra-abdominal sepsis (with an aminoglycoside).

Vancomycin is indicated only in resistant staphylococcal or strep-tococcal endocarditis and in anti-bacterial associated colitis. It is not absorbed orally and causes tissue necrosis on intramuscular injection, and must therefore be given by intravenous infusion. It is bactericidal, and resistance develops rarely. It can cause deafness if the serum concentration is excessive.

Spectinomycin is reserved for the treatment of penicillin-resistant gonorrhoea.

Antibiotics for resistant tuberculosis

If resistance is developed to the standard drugs used for combined therapy one of the following antibiotics can be of value. Synthetic drugs are discussed on page 261.

Rifampicin is bactericidal and highly active against *Myco. tuberculosis* and staphylococci. It is well absorbed orally and is excreted in the bile. Resistance occurs easily and therefore it should be combined with another drug. It is being used increasingly to replace streptomycin in both initial and maintenance therapy. Rifampicin plus isoniazid plus ethambutol is a satisfactory combination for initial treatment, the latter drug being dropped for maintenance therapy. Rifampicin is expensive and this limits it use in developing countries. Although active against staphylococci, it is reserved for use in tuberculosis. It is a potent liver enzyme inducing agent (p. 18).

Capreomycin is a peptide antibiotic whose main action is against the tubercle bacillus. It is ototoxic and nephrotoxic.

Cycloserine is a broad spectrum antibiotic which is useful in tuberculosis as well as in *Esch. coli* and *Proteus* urinary tract infections. It can produce ataxia, drowsiness and convulsions.

Viomycin resembles streptomycin in its antibacterial activity and toxic effects. The latter, however, are much more frequent, and include giddiness, deafness and renal damage. It must be given by injection.

Antileprotic drugs

Dapsone (diaminodiphenylsulphone, DDS) has for many years been the mainstay of treatment of leprosy. It is given orally and treatment may need to be continued for several years. It is well absorbed orally, has a plasma half-life of 20 hours and is largely excreted unchanged in the urine. It is acetylated, like isoniazid (p. 261) and slow acetylators are more susceptible to adverse effects, which include allergic dermatitis, agranulocytosis, methaemoglobinaemia and haemolytic anaemia.

Other drugs used in leprosy include rifampicin (see above), clofazimine (a phenazine dye) and thiambutosine (a diphenylthiourea compound).

Antifungal antibiotics

Although some antibacterial antibiotics, e.g. tetracyclines, have antifungal activity, they are rarely used for this purpose because there are a number of compounds which have specific antifungal activity without much action on bacteria.

Nystatin and amphoterocin B. These are both polyene macrolide antibiotics produced by various *Streptomyces* species. They bind to cell membrane sterols, increasing the permeability of the membrane and causing cell death. Nystatin is used for treating local infections caused by *Candida albicans*. Although it acts against other yeast-like fungi, its toxicity precludes its systemic use. Amphoterocin B, however, is used intravenously for systemic fungal infections, but renal toxicity is prominent. Usually this is reversible, but proliferative changes in the glomeruli may be permanent. Both compounds are poorly soluble and are not well absorbed from the gastrointestinal tract or site of infection. Nystatin is available in various formulations for treating infections of the mouth, alimentary tract, vagina and skin.

Flucytosine (*5-fluorocytosine*) is a synthetic pyrimidine derivative which is converted by cytosine deaminase into 5-fluorouracil which is then incorporated into fungal RNA. It can be used systemically as an alternative to amphoterocin B although it is probably less effective than the latter in *Candida* infections.

Imidazoles. Several compounds are available with a broad spectrum of antifungal activity. They affect ergosterol synthesis and interfere with oxidative enzymes, causing a lethal accumulation of hydrogen peroxide. Ketoconazole is effective systemically when given by mouth and this useful feature is leading to its increased use although its relative postion compared with other drugs has yet to be settled. Miconozole is similar, and is available for parenteral use. Clotrimazole and econazole are available for local application.

Griseofulvin is particularly active against dermatophytes because it is incorporated into the keratin of skin, nails and hair. Treatment may be necessary for up to 2 years in order to eliminate nail infections with *Trichophyton* completely. Its absorption is, unusually, increased when it is taken with meals, but phenobarbitone given concurrently, e.g. for epilepsy, reduces its absorption. It has a plasma half-life of about 36 hours.

Antiviral drugs

The development of clinically-useful antiviral drugs has been slow because of several fundamental problems. Viruses gain entrance to body cells and replicate by distorting normal synthetic processes of the cells. For an agent to suppress viral replication it would first of all have to penetrate into the host cell, and then inhibit the enzymatic processes producing viral nucleic acids and proteins without affecting those of the cell. An even more fundamental difficulty is the fact that the peak rate of growth of the virus is usually over before clinical signs of infection appear, and therefore drug treatment is more suited to prophylaxis than to use in an established infection.

Amantadine blocks the entry of virus particles into cells, but this effect is not powerful. Clinical trials of this compound as a prophylactic drug in influenza have shown variable results, but the duration and severity of the infection seems to be reduced. A more successful application is in the treatment of Parkinsonism (p. 87).

Idoxuridine is a thymidine analogue which inhibits the utilization of thymidine in DNA synthesis. This interferes with the replication of herpes viruses. Continuous topical application of 40% idoxuridine in dimethyl-sulphoxide is effective in skin and eye lesions caused by herpes simplex or varicella zoster virus. It has been little used systemically because of its unacceptable toxicity on the bone marrow, liver and kidneys.

Vidarabine is a purine analogue with activity against herpes viruses; it has a preferential effect on virus as opposed to cellular DNA synthesis. In immunosuppressed patients with shingles it has been shown to reduce pain but its effect is probably small.

Acyclovir is an acyclic nucleoside analogue which is preferentially absorbed by herpes-infected cells where it is phosphorylated by virally specified thymidine kinase into an active substance which inhibits viral DNA polymerase up to 30 times more than cellular DNA polymerase. It is the drug of first choice in severe herpes simplex infections but needs to be given as early as possible after the onset of the illness. It is available for oral, parenteral or local use. It is 30 times less active against varicella zoster virus.

Methisazone inhibits pox viruses at a late stage in their maturation. It is of little value in established smallpox but it has been successfully used as a prophylactic agent in smallpox contacts. It appears also to be of value in reducing the severity of vaccinia when it is given on the fourth day after vaccination of patients who are at special risk, e.g. those with eczematous lesions.

Interferons are highly active glycoproteins which are released by cells invaded by virus particles, probably because the virus induces the production of a messenger RNA which acts as a template for interferons. They probably act on cell membrane receptor sites causing intracellular production of proteins which inhibit the translation of viral messenger RNA. Three types of human interferon exist, leucocyte interferon (obtained from buffy-coat lymphocytes which have been exposed to para-influenza virus), fibroblast interferon (derived from fibroblasts induced with synthetic double-stranded RNA) and 'immune' interferon (derived from T lymphocytes exposed to antigens to which they have been sensitized).

Small quantities of interferon have been made available for trial in virus infections. Promising results have been reported in prophylaxis in immunosuppressed patients, in respiratory infections, viral diseases of the eye, herpes zoster and chronic virus infections such as genital warts. Commercial production of larger quantities will allow further evaluation of this potentially valuable therapeutic substance.

FURTHER READING

Garrod L P, Lambert H P, O'Grady F 1981 Antibiotic and chemotherapy, 5th edn. Churchill Livingstone, Edinburgh

20

Drugs in parasitic infections

Antiprotozoal drugs

An understanding of the treatment of malaria is dependent upon
a knowledge of the life cycle of the causative protozoan, the plasmodium. This is illustrated in Fig. 20.1.

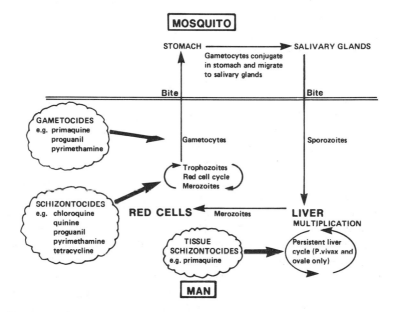

Fig. 20.1 Life cycle of the plasmodium.

There are four types of plasmodium, causing three types of
clinical syndrome. Malignant tertian malaria, the most dangerous
infection, is due to *Plasmodium falciparum* and is most commonly
acquired in tropical Africa. Benign tertian malaria (caused by
P. vivax or *P. ovale*) and quartan malaria (caused by *P. malariae*) are
usually acquired in Asia.

The treatment of malaria has two aspects: treatment of acute infections, and prophylactic therapy.

Treatment of acute infections

The choice of drug depends upon the type of infection. *P. vivax* and *P. ovale* have persistent liver cycles and to establish a 'radical cure' (i.e. totally eliminating the protozoa from the human host) it is necessary to administer a *tissue schizonticide*. Drugs which act only on the red cell cycle (*schizonticides*) will produce only a 'clinical cure' with these types of infection, and subsequent relapse will occur as the liver forms emerge and reinfect the red cells. In contrast, schizonticides will eradicate *P. falciparum* and *P. malariae* infection completely because there are no persistent stages of the parasite in the liver. Some drugs have an additional gametocidal action and will interrupt the life cycle by preventing infection of mosquitoes by the host.

Individual drugs. Chloroquine, a synthetic 4-aminoquinoline, is the drug of choice for treatment of acute attacks (clinical cure) of malaria caused by *P. vivax*, *P. ovale*, *P. malariae* and susceptible strains of *P. falciparum*. It is given orally or intravenously and has a plasma half-life of 120 hours. About 70% is excreted unchanged, the remainder being converted largely to desethylchloroquine. It can cause headache, visual disturbances, pruritis and gastrointestinal upsets. Longer term administration, e.g. for malarial prophylaxis (see below) or rheumatoid arthritis (p. 227), can cause retinopathy, lichenoid skin eruptions, bleaching of hair, diminution of T waves in the ECG and ototoxicity.

Quinine, given orally as the sulphate or intravenously as the dihydrochloride, is the drug of choice in chloroquine-resistant falciparum malaria (sometimes in combination with sulphadoxine and pyrimethamine, or tetracycline). Like chloroquine, it is a 4-aminoquinoline but is naturally occurring in cinchona bark. It is well absorbed orally, is largely metabolized in the liver to hydroxy metabolites and has a plasma half-life of 10 hours. In therapeutic doses it frequently causes mild cinchonism, comprising tinnitus, changes in auditory acuity, headache, blurred vision and nausea. Urticaria, pruritis and asthma can be provoked in susceptible individuals, and haematological toxicity comprising acute haemolysis, hypoprothrombinaemia, thrombocytopenic purpura and agranulocytosis, can occur with larger doses. It has a direct relaxant effect on skeletal muscle and is used to relieve night cramps. Its isomer, quinidine, has antidysrhythmic properties (p. 147).

Proguanil, a biguanide compound, is a folate antagonist acting by inhibition of dihydrofolate reductase. It acts slowly because it has to be converted into active metabolites. Pyrimethamine, a pyrimidine derivative, is closely related chemically to one of the active metabolites of proguanil and has similar dehydrofolate reductase inhibiting properties. It has a plasma half-life of 96 hours. Both drugs have a wider antiplasmodial action than chloroquine, being both schizontocidal and gametocidal. They are often used in combination with dapsone or sulphadoxine in treating chloroquine-resistant falciparium malaria. Their antifolate action can cause haematological, abnormalities which can be reversed by administration of folinic acid (leucovorin). Trimethoprim is closely related to pyrimethamine, and is used as an antibacterial drug (p. 258).

Primaquine is an 8-aminoquinoline used to prevent relapses or provide a radical cure of malaria caused by *P. vivax* or *P. ovale*. It has only tissue schizontocidal and gametocidal activity and is not of value in treating the clinical attack. It is well absorbed orally, is completely metabolized in the liver and has a short plasma half-life. Its major adverse effect is haemolytic anaemia occurring in patients with glucose-6-phosphate dehydrogenase deficiency, particularly of the Mediterrancan variant.

Prophylaxis

Travellers to malarious areas are advised to take prophylactic drug therapy. The choice of drug depends upon the type of plasmodium most likely to be encountered. Chloroquine is a satisfactory choice in areas where the parasites are known to be sensitive to this drug. When chloroquine-resistant species likely to be encountered, combinations of pyrimethamine and dapsone (available as Maloprim) or pyrimethamine and sulphadoxime (Fansidar) are usually selected. Prophylactic therapy is normally started 1–2 weeks before travelling, and continued during and for 4–8 weeks after the visit. Primaquine is sometimes administered following this course for travellers who have been heavily exposed to plasmodia with persistent liver forms.

Drugs for other protozoal diseases

Genito-urinary tract infections with *Trichomonas vaginalis* are common and are usually treated with local or systemic administration of metronidazole or tinidazole. Povidone-iodine can also be used by local application. Gastrointestinal infections with *Enta-*

Table 20.1   Anthelmintic drugs

Drug	Mode of action	Absorption	Excretion	Toxicity	Drug of choice in	Other uses
Pyrantel pamoate	Depolarization of myoneural junction by anticholinesterase effect. Paralysis of worm.	Low	90% faeces 10% urine	Neuromuscular blockade in excess.	*Ascaris* *Enterobius*	Hookworms
Mebendazol	Irreversibly inhibits glucose uptake.	Low	90% faeces 10% urine	None known.	*Trichuris* *Enterobius*	*Ascaris* Hookworms *Enterobius*
Piperazine	Blocks cholinergic receptors. Paralysis of worm.	High	25% metabolised	No serious toxicity.	*Ascaris*	*Enterobius*
Thiabendazole	Unknown. Kills larval and encysted forms.	High	10% faeces 90% urine	Anorexia, nausea dizziness. Hepatotoxic.	*Strongyloides* Cutaneous larva migrans	Hookworms
Bephenium hydroxynaphthoate	Unknown.	No	Faeces	Nausea, vomiting, diarrhoea.	*Ancylostoma*	*Necator*
Tetrachlorethylene	Reversibly paralyses worm. Interferes with intracellular digestive processes.	High	Metabolised	Nausea, vomiting. CNS effects.	*Necator*	
Niclosamide	Interferes with respiration and blocks glucose uptake.	No	Faeces	None known.	All tapeworms	
Antimonials (antimony potassium tartrate and stibophen)	Inhibit phosphofructokinase.	Used parenterally	Urine	Vomiting, renal tubular damage, arthralgia, bone marrow depression, bradycardia. Hepatotoxic.	Schistosomes (*S. mansoni* — stibophen; *S. japonicum* — antimony potassium tartrate)	

Niridazole	Inhibits uptake of exogenous glucose.	Complete	Metabolised	Confusion, convulsions. Flattening of T waves in ECG. Haemolysis in G-6-PD deficient subjects.	Schistosoma haematobium Dracunculus medinensis	S. mansoni S. japonicum
Praziquantel	Unknown	High	Nausea, dizziness	S. mansoni, japonicum, haematobium	Tapeworms	
Diethylcarba-mazine	Unknown. Renders microflariae susceptible to phagocytosis.	High	Urine	Headache, myalgia, athralgia, nausea.	All filariae except Dracunculus medinensis	
Paromomycin	Unknown.	Low	Faeces	Diarrhoea.		Tapeworms
Pyrvinium pamoate	Inhibits oxygen uptake and absorption of exogenous glucose.	No	Faeces	Nausea and vomiting.	Enterobius	

moeba histolytica or *Giardia lamblia* are also effectively managed with metronidazole or tinidazole given by oral administration.

Anthelmintic drugs

Anthelmintic drugs are an assorted group of compounds which share the property of toxicity to parasitic worms. As helmintic infections are amongst the most common of human diseases, they have wide application. A summary of the drugs available, their mode of action and their applications is given in Table 20.1.

For the roundworms, *Enterobius vermicularis* and *Ascaris lumbricoides*, and for the hookworm, *Ancylostoma duodenale*, pyrantel pamoate is an effective drug. In *Enterobius vermicularis* infestations, however, mebendazole is equally effective. Both of these drugs have the advantage that single doses are curative. Infestation with the new world hookworm, *Necator americanus*, is best treated with tetrachlorethylene rather than pyrantel pamoate.

Strongyloides stercoralis, which can become disseminated and can cause recurrent itchy wheals due to migratory larvae, can be eradicated only with thiabendazole therapy. The nematode, *Trichuris trichuria*, is usually eliminated by mebendazole.

When roundworms invade tissues; e.g. visceral larva migrans caused by the dog roundworm *Toxocara canis*, only non-specific therapy such as systemic anti-inflammatory drugs and corticosteroids can be used. In cutaneous larva migrans caused by dog hookworms, however, thiabendazole may destroy the larvae. Only symptomatic therapy can be offered in *Trichinella spiralis* infestations, which can cause severe multisystem inflammatory disease during the migratory phase.

Filarial infections are difficult to manage; diethylcarbamazine is the best available drug, but release of antigens from dead or dying worms may cause systemic reactions which require corticosteroid therapy.

Tapeworms (*Cestodes*) can generally be eliminated by single dose therapy with niclosamide or multi-dose therapy with paromomycin.

Of the fluke infections, those caused by schistosomes are the most serious. Unfortunately, the antimonial compounds used to eliminate *Schistosoma mansoni* and *S. japonicum* are amongst the more toxic of anthelmintic drugs. Niridazole is a drug of first choice in *S. haematobium* infections. A relatively new drug, praziquantel, appears to be effective in infections due to all three main species of schistosomes.

21

Treatment of poisoning

Each year in the United Kingdom approximately 125 000 patients are admitted to hospital because of acute poisoning. Annual deaths from poisoning (excluding carbon monoxide) have remained steady for several years at around 3000, two-thirds of whom die before they reach hospital. The most common causes of poisoning are: accidental, which normally occurs in children aged between 1 and 5 years; and deliberate, as a suicidal attempt or gesture.

Homicidal poisoning and non-accidental poisoning (particularly of children) are much less common, but should not be overlooked.

Whatever the nature of the drug or chemical, the general principles of management are the same.

1. Maintenance of airway and ventilation

Most patients who die of poisoning outside hospital do so because of upper airways obstruction. The airway should, therefore, first be cleared by removing any dentures, pulling the tongue forward and removing saliva and vomitus from the mouth and pharynx. In the deeply unconscious patient with no cough reflex, an endotracheal tube is necessary; in other cases, a short oropharyngeal airway should be inserted. The patient should then be turned to the semi-prone position and the adequacy of ventilation assessed. If there is any suspicion of inadequate ventilation, oxygen should be administered and assisted ventilation considered. In less urgent situations, regular arterial blood gas analysis is the best way to assess ventilation. Analeptic drugs should be avoided, since they may produce convulsions and cardiac arrhythmias.

2. Maintenance of cardiovascular function

Drugs may cause hypotension by a number of mechanisms,

285

including depression of the vasomotor centre and an increase in venous capacitance, leading to reduced venous return to the heart and a consequent fall in cardiac output. If hypotension does not respond to elevation of the foot of the bed, a central venous pressure line should be inserted and colloid (e.g. Haemaccel) infused continuously to increase the intravascular volume. If adequate volume replacement fails to reverse the hypotension, consideration should be given to any possible specific means to remove the toxin (e.g. charcoal haemoperfusion) or inotropic agents (e.g. dopamine or dobutamine).

Cardiac arrhythmias may occur in overdose and contribute to further reduction in cardiac output. Correction of hypoxia or acidosis may abolish arrhythmias, but if not, careful consideration should be given to specific drug therapy, remembering however, that many antiarrhythmic agents may potentiate the negative intropic effects associated with overdose.

3. Control of pain

Intense pain may occur with poisoning from ingestion of corrosive substances. It should be treated with potent analgesics (e.g. morphine).

4. Management of neurological sequelae

Routine care of the unconscious patient should include assessment of the level of consciousness, regular turning to avoid skin damage and nerve and muscle compression injuries. The bladder can often be emptied by firm suprapubic pressure, but catheterization is necessary if this manoeuvre fails, despite marked bladder distension, or when measurement of urine production is important. Cerebral oedema may be caused by hypoxia, hypercapnia, hypoglycaemia or hypotension. It should be carefully looked for in patients who have sustained a cardiorespiratory arrest and should be treated initially with mannitol intravenously, followed by dexamethasone intramuscularly.

Convulsions, if infrequent and of short duration, do not require specific therapy, but can normally be controlled by intravenous diazepam. If the patient is also vomiting, temporary intubation and mechanical ventilation may be necessary to prevent aspiration pneumonia.

5. Identification of the poison

This is important in determining subsequent management. If a reliable history is not available, clinical features and subsequent laboratory investigation may help to identify the toxin(s).

6. Reduction of absorption

Gastric lavage (or induced emesis) may reduce further absorption of drug. It is indicated in poisoning with dangerous compounds when the time of ingestion is unknown or with 4 hours of known ingestion. Certain drugs (e.g. salicylates, opiates, anticholinergic drugs and tricyclic antidepressants) delay gastric emptying and lavage or emesis may be effective later than 4 hours. In the unconscious patient, a cuffed endotracheal tube must always be inserted before lavage is instituted. Lavage and emesis are contraindicated in poisoning with corrosive agents, unless the danger of systemic toxicity is greater than the risk of oesophageal perforation (e.g. as with concentrated paraquat or formic acid). Lavage and emesis are also contraindicated after oral ingestion of petroleum distillates because of the risk of aspiration pneumonia.

Emesis (normally with syrup of ipecacuanha) is unlikely to be effective after antiemetic poisoning and should not be performed in the patient whose consciousness is impaired.

Oral adsorbents (e.g. activated charcoal) may be of value, particularly in accidental poisoning in children, since they normally present early enough for the adsorbent to be effective.

7. Enhancement of drug elimination

Forced diuresis increases the renal clearance of salicylates, phenobarbitone and phenoxyacetate herbicides (e.g. 2.4D) when the urine is alkaline, and amphetamines, fenfluramine and phencyclidine when the urine is acid.

Such patients should have normal cardiac and renal function since the diuresis is achieved by infusing large volumes of fluid intravenously. A careful assessment of fluid balance is therefore necessary, and unconscious patients require bladder catheterization. If the fluid input exceeds the output at any stage by 2 litres or more, intravenous frusemide is given. The aim of alkaline diuresis is to maintain the urine pH between 7.0 and 8.0 (checked by indicator paper) but if large amounts of bicarbonate are needed to achieve this, the arterial pH and serum potassium and calcium should be carefully monitored. Forced acid diuresis is less frequently required. Ammonium chloride is given (either orally or intravenously) to keep urine pH below 5.0 and careful monitoring of arterial pH is also mandatory. Haemodialysis is useful in removing drugs which have low plasma protein binding, volume of distribution and lipid solubility. It is generally reserved for treatment of severe overdosage, particularly in those patients with secondary complications. Salicylates, phenobarbitone, ethanol, methanol and lithium are effectively removed by this method. Haemoperfusion of arterial blood through an extracorporeal column of activated charcoal or ion-exchange resin will effectively remove some drugs, even though their lipid solubility and/or plasma protein binding may be high. It is again reserved for severe poisoning, particularly when serious complications are present. Barbiturates, glutethimide, methaqualone, ethchlorvynol, meprobamate, chloral hydrate and theophylline may be effectively removed by this method.

Specific measures

In a few instances, specific measures may be indicated in addition to the general measures already discussed.

Opiates

Naloxone is effective in reversing the respiratory and cardiovascular depression seen in opiate overdose. Such agents include cough suppressants (e.g. dextromethorphan), anti-diarrhoeal agents (diphenoxylate), as well as analgesics (e.g. pentazocine and dextropopoxyphene). It is only partially effective in reversing the effects of buprenorphine and may have to be given by intravenous infusion to reverse the effects of the longer acting opiates (e.g. methadone).

Cyanide

The inhalation of hydrogen cyanide usually causes death within a few minutes, but after oral ingestion, symptoms may occur later. Dicobalt edetate intravenously is the treatment of choice. Subsequent gastric lavage with sodium thiosulphate is also indicated after oral ingestion.

Heavy metals

After oral ingestion of large amounts of metallic salts, lavage should be performed and chelating agents should be used. Dimercaprol is effective in arsenic, mercury and gold poisoning, calcium disodium edetate in lead poisoning, desferrioxamine in iron poisoning, Prussian blue in thallium poisoning and penicillamine in copper poisoning.

Methanol and ethylene glycol

Ethanol administration (oral or intravenous) reduces the metabolism of these agents to toxic intermediate compounds and thus reduces toxicity.

Paracetamol

Overdosage with paracetamol, can produce hepatic necrosis and renal failure. Plasma paracetamol concentration should be measured, and if the value is greater than shown in Figure 21.1 at any particular time, acetylcysteine should be given by intravenous infusion. If more than 8 hours have elapsed after ingestion of more than 7.5 G, acetylcysteine, which repletes glutathione stores and allows conjugation of the toxic intermediate metabolite to form a harmless conjugate, should be given immediately and the subsequent plasma paracetamol concentration used as a guide to whether the therapy should be continued. Oral methionine is also effective up to 10 hours after overdose if the patient is not vomiting (which often happens in severe paracetamol poisoning). Early paracetamol concentrations may be falsely low due to delayed gastric emptying caused by other drugs taken concurrently (e.g. dextropropoxyphene in 'Distalgesic'). Enzyme-inducing drugs may predispose to toxicity by increasing the rate of formation of the hepatotoxic metabolite and treatment may be indicated if the paracetamol concentration is 70% or more of the levels shown in Fig. 21.1

Cholinesterase inhibitors

These agents are found most often in the form of organophosphorus insecticides and many produce prolonged signs associated with excessive acetycholine accumulation at nerve endings. Atropine may antagonize the muscarinic effects and oximes (pralidoxime) will reactivate cholinesterase if given within the first 12 hours.

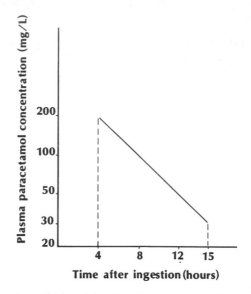

Fig. 21.1 Line above which acetylcysteine therapy for paracetamol poisoning should be given.

Paraquat

This weedkiller is corrosive, but also causes severe systemic pulmonary and renal toxicity. Fuller's Earth (or bentonite) bind the compound in the gut, but must be given early (within 6 hours) to be effective.

Aspirin

Acute overdose may lead to restlessness, tinnitus, deafness, hyperthermia, dehydration, respiratory alkalosis and metabolic acidosis. This may be associated with hypokalaemia, hypopothrombinaemia and, more rarely, pulmonary oedema and acute renal failure. Coma is a late and very serious prognostic feature. Forced alkaline diuresis may be useful if the plasma level is greater than 450 mg/l and haemodialysis or haemoperfusion may be indicated if the plasma level exceeds 1000 mg/l.

Digoxin

Overdose causes nausea, vomiting, confusion, diarrhoea, hyperkalaemia and cardiac arrhythmias. Hyperkalaemia may need treatment with dialysis if severe, and bradyarrhythmias may require a transvenous pacemaker to be inserted temporarily. In severe cases specific Fab antibody administration may reduce toxicity. Consult the National Poisons Information Service for advice on its availability (Table 21.1).

Table 21.1 National Poisons Information Service

Belfast	(0232) 240503
Cardiff	(0222) 569200
Dublin	(0001) 745588
Edinburgh	(031) 229-2477
London	(01) 635-9191
or	(01) 407-7600
Other Centres	
Birmingham	(021) 554-3801
Leeds	(0532) 430715
Newcastle	(0632) 325131

FURTHER READING

Proudfoot A 1982 Diagnosis and management of acute poisoning. Blackwell Scientific Publications, Oxford
Vale J A, Meredith T J 1985 A concise guide to the management of poisoning. Churchill Livingstone, Edinburgh

Index